ALSO BY JOHN BLADE

The Bitcoin Capital of the World

Weight Chaining

Total Body Fat Incinerator

Pandemic Armor

EXERLEAN

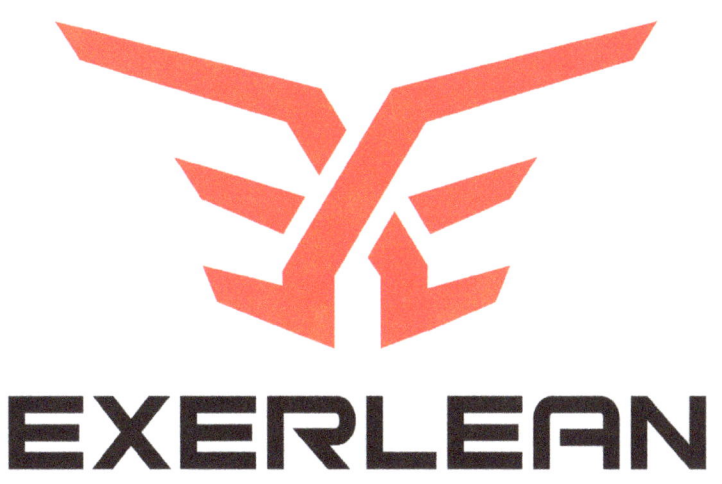

EXERLEAN

Resolution for the Physique Transformation of a Lifetime

Get Lean

Get Strong

Get Healthy

JOHN BLADE

Praise for John Blade and EXERLEAN

"John's career as an occupational therapist and lifelong love of health and wellness has given him a perspective worth noting. His ideas may just get you the fitness level you dream of if you get off the couch and give them a try."

—Mary A. J.
PharmD

"John Blade is truly authentic in his articulation of the human body when it comes to fitness and dieting in this book. His achievments in real estate, bodybuilding, wall street, and as an Occupational Therapist marks a man that is driven to excellence. His passion to share his knowledge on physique transformation is apparent. This book is a must read for those willing to do the work necessary to attain new heights of physical bad-assness and quality of life."

—Daniel J. Nickel
COTA

"EXERLEAN delivers the goods. As the author writes, "hold on to your saddlebags" you better suit up your armor for this one. This approach to weight loss and health transformation is likely the end answer in the quest for the obesity cure."

—Elizabeth K.
PharmD

"This book really motivated me to begin a weight loss plan, to start exercising daily, and to stick with it. John Blade presents the case in a way that leaves no wiggle room for escape from the inevitable. Do it or die! EXERLEAN is the way."
—Anne Hogue.

Client

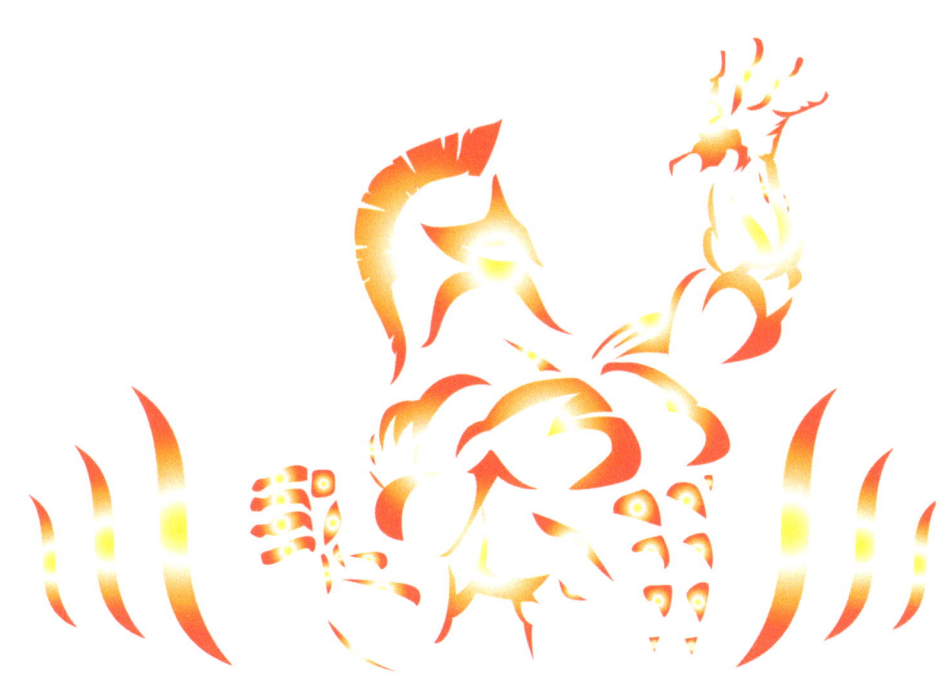

EXERLEAN™
Copyright © 2021 John Blade. All rights reserved.

This book or any part thereof may not be reproduced or transmitted in any form or by any means without permission in writing from the authors.

This book is directed toward people without medical complications, diseases, or disabilities. It is not intended to replace professional medical or diet advice. Any use of the information in this book is at the reader's discretion. The author disclaims any specific information contained in this book. Please consult your healthcare professional for medical advice or before starting a diet or exercise regimen.

The author has not been compensated in any manner to promote any products or companies in this book. All products and companies mentioned herein are for informational purposes only.

All Scripture quotations taken from the New American Standard Bible® (NASB),
copyright © 1960, 1962, 1963, 1968, 1971, 1972, 1973, 1975, 1977, 1995 by the Lockman Foundation.
Used by permission. www.lockman.org.

Cover design: George Stevens G Sharp Design LLC
Book design: John Blade

LCCN : 2021922871

ISBN 979-8-88502-000-8 (Hardcover)
ISBN 979-8-88502-002-2 (paperback)
ISBN 979-8-88502-001-5 (e-book)
ISBN 979-8-88502-003-9 (Audiobook)

Printed in the United States of America

www.exerlean.com

To all those who have requested my assistance to lose weight and get in better shape.

Now is your time.

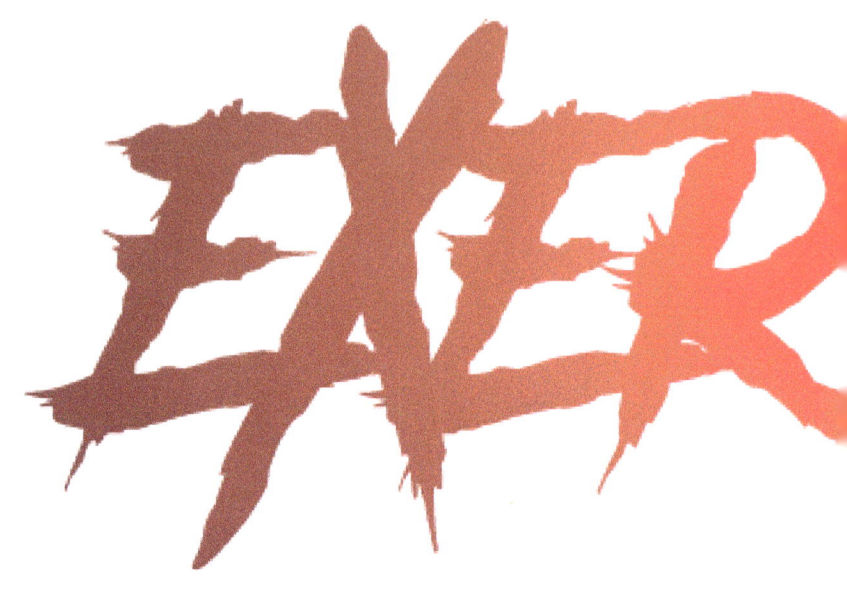

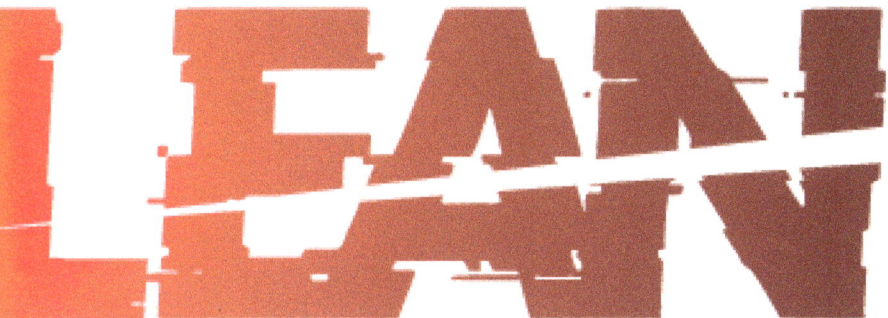

"Some people want it to happen. Some wish it would happen. Others make it happen."

Michael Jordan

"If you have discipline, drive, and determination... Nothing is impossible."
Dana Linn Bailey

"We must suffer from one of two pains: the pain of discipline or the pain of regret. The discipline weighs ounces while the regret weighs tons."
Jim Rohn

"We can't become what we need to be by remaining what we are."
Oprah Winfrey

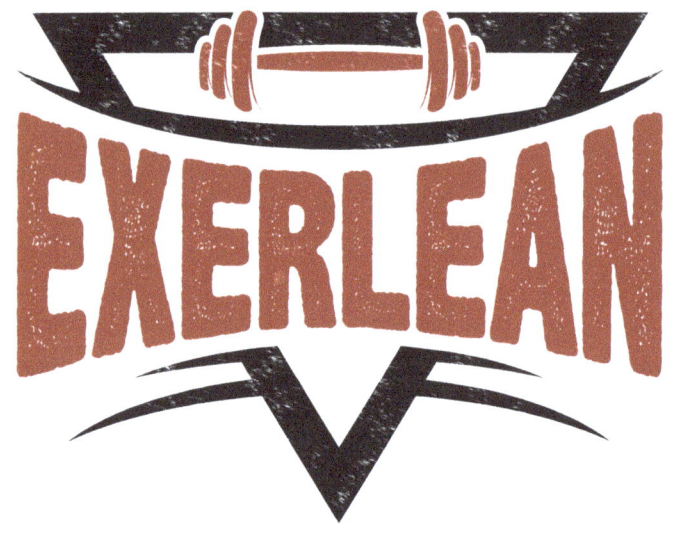

Before we begin your transformation journey . . .

This book has been put together to reprogram your mind. To alter your perception of body fat and obesity, dieting, exercise, and weight training. To help you change your self-destructive mindset and replace it with one that is productive, motivated, and primed for a successful transformation. To help you change your behavior, which may be the reason you're in the predicament, whatever it is, that you are in. To help you slay your enemies, whatever entities they are, and stop them from incapacitating you and your hopes of achieving a healthy and lean body.

Beginning to end, every element of the book is laid out with strategic purpose and order. It is vital to enter this journey open-minded and ready—in fact, motivated and yearning—for change. To have a successful transformation, you must do the work. Everybody must start somewhere. The first step toward a goal must be taken to achieve transformation. The first step is to read this book from the first word to the last. Do not skip or read out of order.

There are times in this book you may feel overwhelmed, hammered, exhausted, and doubtful. You will review intimate, personal, and deeply troubling areas of life. Everything is raw, real, and necessary. Negative reinforcement leads to positive reinforcement and reprogramming. After all, you cannot prevent the bad you are unaware of. The negative side effects of being overweight, obese, or morbidly obese are fully disclosed to help you prevent them from entering your life or extinguish them if already present.

Stay focused, open-minded, and willing to change the way you view things. If the best things in life were comfortable and easy to attain, we would all be rich, lean, and in perfect health. Right!

Like the buildup of a good plot in your favorite fiction book, the end delivers the goods. You will walk away from this book with all the right stuff—fully prepared for your ultimate physique transformation, adopting positive habits, and living a life of health and wellness.

Contents

Introduction 1

Part 1: Wakie Wakie...Slap your Facie. 3
    Chapter 1: The Face Slap 5
    Chapter 2: The Obesiboomers 9
    Chapter 3: Why Change? 13
    Chapter 4: Wipe Your Own! 21
    Chapter 5: Dadbodinator 35
    Chapter 6: Bodinomics: The Economy of the Human Body 49
    Chapter 7: Bodinomics: Fuel 55
    Chapter 8: Bodinomics: Work 59
    Chapter 9: Healthstyle 63

Part 2: The "EXER" in EXERLEAN 75
    Chapter 10: EXERLEAN 77
    Chapter 11: The Benefits of Exercise 81
    Chapter 12: Weight Training 89
    Chapter 13: Weight Chaining 111
    Chapter 14: Fasted Cardio 123
    Chapter 15: EXERPAIN 127

Part 3: The "LEAN" in EXERLEAN 135
    Chapter 16: Bodinomics: Nutrition 137
    Chapter 17: How to Get Fat 149
    Chapter 18: Low-Glycemic Carbohydrates 163
    Chapter 19: High Biological Value (BV) Proteins 173
    Chapter 20: The State 181
    Chapter 21: Supplementation 217

Part 4: Execute & Launch 221
   Chapter 22: Putting It All Together 223
   Chapter 23: Preparation + Execution + Launch! 227
   Chapter 24: Lean Tools 231
   Chapter 25: EXERBAG: Your Gym Bag Essentials 247
   Chapter 26: Phase One: Cutting 251
   Chapter 27: Phase Two: Maintenance 255
   Chapter 28: The Final Chapter: Not the End but the Beginning ..265

Bonus: 12 Dieting Facts 267

Bonus: KISS Tips 269

Glossary 271

References 273

Other Resources 285

Referrals 287

About the Author 289

Introduction

BEHOLD THE DAWN of a new age. The age of a new and better you destined for a life of maximal health and wellness. An age where you take control of your actions, your body, your behavior, and your habits. Let this book be your source of motivation. Your stun gun and trigger point to propel you toward improved self-care, self-help, and optimal quality of life.

Herein lies the answers, the resources, and the plan to achieve your best you. To learn and earn ultimate success in annihilating your mortal enemies—body fat and sedentary death.

EXERLEAN gives you the keys to the car and puts you in the cockpit. The material within will help you steer through life in the right direction. To help you achieve your vision and goals for body composition, quality of life, and maximal health and wellness. Minus the wasted time and angst a person goes through with fake diets, fad diets, celebrity diets, bug diets, juice diets, yo-yo diets, no diets, food confusion, and the never-ending body weight fluctuations.

The truth is hard at times, but the truth is exactly what is necessary to devise a plan that will achieve *real* results. The truth, the *raw* truth, and that's exactly what will be delivered to you in this book, straight up! Hold the bullshit.

Grab on, hold on tight, and don't let go!

Let's begin the journey.

PART I

Wakie Wakie...Slap your Facie.

CHAPTER 1
The Face Slap

ARE YOU SICK and tired of living unhealthy, feeling like a low-energy pile of crap, and never being able to see beyond the fat on your body every time you look in the mirror? Well, look no further because this book, right here in your hands, has everything necessary to help you put an end to excess body fat and the negative consequences that come with it.

Before you read any further, I want to warn you that this book is a slap-in-the-face, no-holds-barred, possibly-some-bad-words *awakening*.

An awakening to the reality of the world around you and why the majority of people are overweight, sedentary, and in some cases, dying earlier than they should. You may be one of them!

Okay, now . . . if you're complaining, then pull up your big-boy or big-girl pants and accept that you may be part of the worldwide obesity epidemic.

Hold on to your saddlebags! We are about to take a ride down reality lane.

"Let's Do This!"

Two out of three adult human beings are considered overweight, obese, or morbidly obese as of 2018 per the National Institutes of Health (NIH). Per 2013–2014 NHANES (National Health and Nutrition Examination Survey) data, **70.2 percent of adults are overweight or obese, 32.5 percent are overweight, and 37.7 percent are obese, of which 7.7 percent includes extreme obesity**. Additionally, **three out of four men** (73.7 percent) and **two out of three women** (66.9 percent) are considered overweight, obese, or morbidly obese. Sadly, **one in six youth** ages two to nineteen (17.2 percent) were considered to be obese (NHANES Data, NIH).

Now I'm not saying you're overweight, but your chances of being overweight or obese are overwhelming. Most of us are overweight at the minimum. In fact, unless you have been on and are currently undergoing some sort of exercise routine and have been eating lean, then you are at a minimum overweight and possibly obese.

So, from here forward knowing that over 70 percent of us are overweight, obese, or morbidly obese, we have a literally big problem on our hands. Unless you're in the less than 30 percent of people maintaining a healthy weight, then you desperately need to take everything this book has to offer, cram it down your throat, and live it out.

Let the awareness of the obesity epidemic move you toward a positive change. To help you on your journey to lose weight, get strong, and learn and adopt healthy, lean living habits.

I call this a transformation of a person's *healthstyle*. Lifestyle includes everything about you and how you're living—your car, job, hobbies, religion, beliefs, morals, activities, routines, schedules, health, exercise, etc. Your healthstyle includes everything you engage in mentally, physically, leisurely, and workwise that actually and factually dictates your current state of body composition, health, and wellness.

Moving forward, we are going to talk about some possibly shocking, personal, and revealing details about humanity that may initially offend you, maybe humiliate you, possibly upset you. But fear not—there is a greater mission than that at hand.

After assimilating the knowledge, statistics, and resources this book offers, the goal is that you will become externally influenced and internally motivated for positive change. To change your ways, to stake your claim on this earth and make your life the best it can be.

> **"Anything can happen if you make a move.
> Nothing different will if you don't."** —Me

In 2004, while in the school of occupational therapy (OT) at Eastern Washington University (EWU), I wrote a research paper and grant application to the National Institutes of Health titled, "Does Obesity Affect a Person's Occupational Performance in Community Mobility?" The results of my study were staggering. One of the first things I became aware of from my research was the exponential rising prevalence of obesity in America, especially in children. As to my research title's question, the overwhelming statistics and data reveal the answer is a huge yes. Sadly, obesity does negatively affect a person's ability to mobilize within their community and the quality of their mobilization. For example, these problems could include requirements to pay for two airplane seats due to buttocks width, use of power scooters for shopping, inaccessibility through standard-width doorways, higher-priced furniture and medical equipment to handle the excess weight, and difficulty getting on and maneuvering public buses or subway systems. The list goes on and on and on.

Sadly, since I did that research at OT school in 2004, the obesity epidemic is only growing exponentially out of control. Straight to who knows where. At the rate that body fat is increasing in the United States, we are headed toward a 100 percent overweight and obese population.

Why the trend?

What's the reason for the epidemic of overweight people?

CHAPTER 2
The Obesiboomers

What we are seeing and dealing with all started with the silent generation of the early 1900s, specifically 1925 to 1942 during the ramping up of automotive technology and air travel. This is when the flash flood of market-to-consumer products began. High-tech luxuries to make our lives easier. Cars, motorcycles, airplanes, and public transportation systems. No more horses, walking, or riding bikes as a necessity.

The baby boomers' post–World War II generation from about 1940 to 1964 on to Generation X of 1960 to 1981 to the millennial generation and now Generation Z have all reaped the exponentially accumulating benefits of scientific and industrial breakthroughs. We are now living in the splendor and bliss of the technological age. The environment around us makes this undeniable! We are living in the easiest, least physically demanding, most plentiful, and most accessible time in human history.

Easy access to foods, drinks, transportation, and sedentary work environments are at an all-time high and rising with the continual advances in science and technology. And with it, we as a human race have become overweight, obese, and sedentary. Welcome to the dawn of the Obesiboomers!

It's undeniable that we as humans are in a booming phase in the evolution of our species, similar to the massive spike in baby births mid-twentieth century that gave rise to the term *baby boomers*. Well, our species is undergoing a massive transformation into the nether realm of obesity, obesity-related diseases, and obesity-related disabilities. The Obesiboomer epidemic is not specific to one generation, race, or county. Obesity does not discriminate. It is a trend involving the majority of the world. With rates of three out of four U.S. adults being either overweight or obese, the odds are in favor of 70 percent of all people around you being overweight or obese, including yourself. As I said earlier, one in six children are obese, a trend that is only rising and showing no signs of a downtrend or stabilization. This leads in only one direction as we head into the future. A surge in the Obesiboomer epidemic.

The Walt Disney movie *WALL·E* paints a great vision into the future of mankind and how technology may become so advanced that machines will do everything for us. If you haven't seen the movie, I highly recommend watching it as soon as you can. It is a rewarding film for all ages. To sum up the part I am referring to, basically humans live in an automated community on the massive spaceship the *Axiom*. The *Axiom* is so automated that the residents don't even have to walk. They float everywhere they need to go in little hover chairs, enjoying food in overabundance and entertainment galore. They are extremely sedentary, and consequently, everybody is morbidly obese.

This could be the future of the human race if sedentary human behavior becomes the norm and technological advancements keep simplifying our ability to work or not work.

The Obesiboomer millennia is birthed from an environment of less and less physical work. We as a human race are engaging in less and less physically exerting activity as technology makes our lives easier. To fix this dilemma, we need to add in physical work or exercise to compensate for the lack of exertion taking place. The human body needs physical work, exertion, and weight-bearing activity every day to maintain skeletal integrity, muscle functions, and body composition.

Bones need bone-on-bone pressure and weight-bearing activity to stay strong, otherwise sedentary behavior and lack of that pressure will lead to bone demineralization, decreased bone density, mechanical destabilization, and possible structural deformity over time.

Muscles need work and force to maintain mass and strength. Lack of necessary workload on muscles leads to the pruning of muscle tissue and muscle atrophy. This muscle wasting in turn leads to weaker muscle functions, low energy, and lower metabolism.

Without daily workload, our body composition (the balance or ratio between muscles, body fat/adipose tissue, and bone) is distorted away from our natural healthy state of being. Body fat increases, lean body tissue or muscle decreases, and bones become smaller and frail. Add to that, if we are not physically active doing something, then we must consequently be doing nothing—likely sitting in a chair, reading this book, or watching television. Then, human behavior, boredom, and bad habits take over; we grab a snack and start eating garbage at the same time we're being sedentary. This leads to even more body fat storage.

You know the story.

Obesity is preventable and treatable. The chapters to come will provide you with all the right information you need to take control of yourself and your actions.

To take a stand against sedentary behavior and the overstuffing of our faces. To get out of the fat race.

CHAPTER 3
Why Change?

BEFORE WE GET into the secrets on how to change your ways, your health, and your body composition, we first need to fully understand the why.

Why change?

I mean, what's so bad about being overweight or obese? It's the new norm, it's accepted, and as time goes by, it's universally rationalized or even normalized as beautiful and healthy. Nobody really cares if you're overweight or obese.

What does it matter?

Is media and societal-driven propaganda coaxing or forcing us to accept being overweight or obese as normal, beautiful, or good?

I've never heard someone say that "her folds of fat and cratered cellulite legs are really flattering." or "Oh, boy, he's got an attractive, bulbous potbelly."

I mean, come on, let's stick to reality here. You'd be living a lie if you said or tried to convince yourself that folds of fat, dimply legs, or protruding potbellies were attractive, preferred, or normal compared to a slender, muscular, or lean physique.

"Come on, everyone's doing it."

Does a societal norm make something a good thing just because the majority are experiencing it, like obesity?

Yeah, let's all jump off the cliff.

If it's not good, then it must be bad, and if it's bad . . . how bad? How bad is being overweight, obese, or morbidly obese . . . really?

Okay, well, where do we start? Let's start with this: the most up-to-date information from the NIH and the Centers for Disease Control and Prevention (CDC). Obesity and obesity-related diseases lead to early death.

Death!

Yes, dead before your time. In other words, people who are not overweight or obese stand a much greater chance at longevity than fat people. Add to this, the last decade or two of life is of much lower quality for obese or morbidly obese persons. This is due to their poor health status, poor ability to self-care, joint destruction, poor mobility, and onset of and living with obesity-related diseases and disabilities.

I have worked as an occupational therapist (OT) since 2004 in the acute care hospital setting with direct patient care. I'm the guy who comes into a patient's room and helps them get out of bed, mobilize, and engage in self-care. OTs focus on helping people rehabilitate from surgery, illness, disease, or disability. We do this by facilitating their engagement in self-care and mobility, as well as quality of life. We initiate exercises or therapeutic activities to get people up and moving so they can take care of themselves and return to their home.

I've helped thousands of patients rehabilitate and continue to do so full time. As an OT in an acute care hospital setting, I see everything. I work with people going through negative life events including intubation on a ventilator in the intensive care unit (ICU), strokes and heart attacks, pneumonia, falls with injury, trauma from motor vehicle accidents, and respiratory failure. I bounce all over the hospital, from the oncology unit to cardiac to the ER to the mental health ward and the surgical unit. My job is to teach people how to live after a neck, back, hip, knee, or any other surgery.

I've seen thousands of different diseases, disabilities, trauma situations, and other various physical or mental defects and intervene to help people deal with these problems so they can recover, take care of themselves, and move on in their lives. Much of the stuff people live with is truly unbelievable.

As Winston from the original *Ghostbusters* movie put it, "I've seen shit that will turn you white!"

Healthcare workers see firsthand how people deal with and recover from sickness, disease, or traumatic events. Ask any acute care therapist or nurse, and they will tell you that morbid obesity is one of the most disabling and unhealthy states of human existence. It affects absolutely everything in a negative way.

In order to develop the inner power necessary to make real physical, mental, and lifestyle changes, you need to know the *why*. The knowledge of why gives you the power to change. Then you can enter the battle against obesity. You need to have full knowledge of why you're in the fight against obesity, why body fat is your enemy, and why your life depends on winning the war.

The truth behind being overweight or obese is much more involved than just people being larger, having health problems, and likely dying earlier than expected. The obvious and well-publicized *negative effects* of obesity are prevalent.

Here is a summary of obesity-related data taken from the CDC website: "People who have obesity, compared to those with a normal or healthy weight, are at increased risk for many serious diseases and health conditions, including the following:"

Wait, let's stop there for a second. Before going into the details of these negative effects, I want to point out that government entities like the CDC, universities, and other research entities use very careful language and water down the verbiage to speak about the effects of obesity, choosing words like "are at increased risk," "associated with obesity," "may contribute." I will tell you straight up based on my years of clinical experience and treating people with obesity that obese people absolutely experience and endure more diseases, disabilities, and serious health conditions than lightweight lean people. Some deal with a few too many afflictions at the same time.

Based on clinical observations, the older an obese person gets, the more diseases, health problems, and disabilities just keep piling up like a stack of pancakes. The next thing they know, they are suffering from multiple major issues, which greatly decreases their quality of life. Unfortunately, most obese people choose to deal with these negative effects rather than do anything to combat them.

So let us keep the language real. The CDC's list of obesity-related health disparities include:

All causes of death (mortality). Yes, death means dead. Obesity leads to dead people, or being dead sooner than later.

High blood pressure. Hypertension can quietly destroy your body, leading to strokes, blood clots, dementia, heart attacks, heart and kidney disease, anxiety, poor quality of life, disability, and even fatality. There it is again, death!

High LDL cholesterol (the bad cholesterol), low HDL cholesterol (the good cholesterol), and high levels of triglycerides (bad). Too much bad cholesterol leads to strokes, heart disease, peripheral artery disease (PAD), and various other health ailments. Not enough of the good cholesterol leads to heart disease, digestion problems, and other health ailments.

Coronary heart disease. The heart is the core of all things blood. It is the only pump in the body. When the pumping stops . . . life stops. Heart disease is the most common cause of death for adults in the US. A diseased heart or circulatory system leads to heart failure, heart attack, stroke, pulmonary embolism, aneurysm, peripheral artery disease, heart arrythmias, angina, and lower quality of life.

Type 2 diabetes. Don't blow this one off, it's horrible! Type 2 diabetes increases a person's risk of leg, finger, or hand amputations and of developing low vision, peripheral neuropathy (brain and spinal cord nerve damage), and kidney failure. This can lead to dependency on dialysis machines to live.

Gallbladder disease. Gallbladder disease involves abdominal pain, nausea and vomiting, and infections that can lead to needing surgery to remove the gallbladder—a high-risk surgery.

Osteoarthritis. Osteoarthritis is the breakdown of cartilage and bone within a joint. When you're walking around in public, you'll observe many obese people whose knees are bent inward and are touching each other. Many overweight and obese people have deformed knees and hips because our joints are not designed to handle all that excess weight, and as a result, they will fall apart and disintegrate over time without exercise. This leads to needing joint replacement surgery or living in pain, thus eventually becoming immobile and dependent on power scooters and wheelchairs.

Sleep apnea and breathing problems (drowning in fat). Don't overlook this one! I see it every day in the hospital. Many obese and morbidly obese people have to wear a CPAP (continuous positive airway pressure) or BiPAP (bilevel positive airway pressure) breathing-assist device to keep their airways opened because they are blocked by fat tissues. These people cannot tolerate lying in a normal bed, so the head of the bed needs to be elevated or propped up so they won't suffocate or drown in their own body mass.

Some cancers. All cancer is bad, and you should make every effort to decrease your risk of getting it.

Dementia. Studies have shown that high levels of belly fat are linked to higher levels of brain atrophy (shrinking brains) and dementia. According to a 2008 Massachusetts General Hospital study, heavier people have smaller brains. Obese people were found to have 8 percent smaller-than-average brains and also looked sixteen years older. It also found that people with the most belly fat between the ages of forty and forty-five are three times more likely than normal-weight people to develop dementia in their later years.

Low quality of life (QOL). Of all the negative effects of obesity, except for maybe increased risk of death, this one cannot be understated.

As we live out our existence, it is in our nature to seek out our best quality of life. Obesity is a detrimental weapon working against you on this journey. Long-term obesity leads to poor quality of life. Based on my clinical observations and working firsthand to help people living with obesity, it is never a good thing. I have never witnessed a benefit of obesity in my practice.

People living with obesity get accustomed to it and lose track of the difference between living with a healthy body weight and being heavy. They forget about being able to walk for miles, sitting in one airplane seat, being able to walk down the aisle of a bus without their thighs bouncing off each seat they pass, or walking straight through a narrow doorway versus having to go through sideways. This list is never-ending. All aspects of human life are negatively affected by obesity.

Stroke. We all know strokes are bad and can be disabling. As an OT, I work with victims of strokes and help them return to independent self-care and functional mobility. I help people strengthen the weak body parts affected by the stroke, and I help them return to their best possible lives.

Trust me on this one—obese and morbidly obese people with strokes are usually much worse off than a lightweight stroke victim. Unless it's a minor stroke or a stoke that clears fast, obese people are screwed. Not only do they lose half their body function, but the remaining unaffected overweight side of the body has to carry around its weight and all the weight of the overweight paralyzed side. Add to that, most people with obesity live sedentary lives and are therefore deconditioned in the first place.

Nurses and therapists working with obese and morbidly obese people have their work cut out for them. They are at high risk of injury due to the excess burden of care an obese person requires. In many cases, nurses and therapists must use power cranes to move obese people in and out of bed to a commode or wheelchair. On the contrary, nonobese people are lighter and work less to self-care and mobilize, even with severe stroke deficits. Lightweight people have a much better chance of being able to get in and out of bed or transfer with caregiver assistance and without a crane.

Obese people in the hospital require heavy-duty specialty beds, wheelchairs, and bedside chairs to hold their weight. It's much more expensive, time consuming, and difficult to care for an obese or morbidly obese person compared to a healthy-weight person in the hospital setting. Many obese stroke sufferers end up in nursing homes for the rest of their lives. Healthy and lighter-weight people have much better odds of being able to return home or move to a lesser-care environment than a nursing home.

Family including spouses have a much better chance at being able to help you at home or take care of you if you are healthy and lightweight. Many patients and their families cannot afford the heavy-duty equipment necessary to care for obese and morbidly obese people. In many cases, they are forced to quit their jobs so they can be at home all the time to meet an obese person's higher-care needs. This is one of the reasons nursing homes have a high prevalence of obese residents. Most families cannot handle all that massive weight, give up their jobs, afford the heavy-duty furniture, or give up all their time to care for obese people with severe disability.

There is no going back. The ability to exercise is greatly diminished after a stroke with obesity, and therefore the ability to exercise and lose weight is more difficult. Restrictive dieting is basically the only option at this point, and I can tell you straight up that I've never seen a morbidly obese person with a disability change their behavior and diet to lose all that extra weight to make self-care and mobility easier, not one case in sixteen years. A lifetime of bad eating behavior is not easy to break, although it is absolutely possible. If you are obese, the time to take action is now, not later. Do it now before you stroke out!

Mental illness. Mental illness includes clinical depression, anxiety, and other mental disorders. If you had to live with half the stuff mentioned so far, how could you remain truly happy? We have the power to control how we feel, yes, but you must admit, these ailments would be very difficult to live with twenty-four hours a day and remain mentally unscathed, not to even mention the dissatisfaction with your appearance.

Body pain. What I predominantly see in my practice is that obese people have a much higher prevalence of spine, hip, knee, and ankle pain. Almost all obese people deal with cellulitis, a predicament when their skin gets infected and starts blowing up with puss-oozing fluids. Cellulitis is highly painful and hypersensitive. It usually requires antibiotics to treat. Not all, but most patients with fibromyalgia that I have come in contact with are overweight or obese. Fibromyalgia is another painful infliction.

Now here's where we are going to get down to the nitty-gritty, the behind-the-scenes situations that healthcare workers see firsthand:

How obesity affects personal care.

CHAPTER 4
Wipe Your Own!

ET'S CUT TO the chase and reveal the stuff people don't talk about when it comes to obesity. The most personal and intimate areas of our lives that are taboo to discuss. Personal to the core.

In addition to all the health problems we've mentioned, obesity and especially morbid obesity negatively affect personal self-care. Some obvious effects include difficulty getting in and out of bed, decreased walking distance, difficulty climbing up and down stairs, struggling to get in and out of a car, decreased productivity at work or inability to work, lower energy, and on and on. You can't push a marble through a pinhole.

We never openly discuss our personal abilities to self-care. Think about it. When is the last time you talked to someone about the quality of your ability to brush your teeth or cut your toenails? When's the last time you talked about the quality of your bathing and ability to reach every nook and cranny? "Hey, Bertha! Are you able to get your socks and shoes on these days?" Conversations like this just don't happen openly until self-care is an issue.

It's weird to think that people have difficulty with self-care. For the geriatric population, this is expected at some point as the body ages, becomes frail, and eventually closes in on the end of its days.

Self-care can also be challenging for those with disability from congenital or birth defects, traumatic disability, and injury from accident or other trauma. These issues are accidental and sometimes unpreventable. What we are talking about here is people who are afflicted with the preventable state of being overweight, obese, and morbidly obese.

As we discussed earlier, healthcare workers see thousands and thousands of people daily, many living with obesity and in desperate situations of self-care failure. Much of what they see in the hospital would turn you white, ghost white! They know firsthand the raw truth about how obesity affects people's ability to take care of themselves.

If you're not a nurse, therapist, doctor, or other medical team member, then you're likely just seeing obese people from their outside appearance, walking around, dressed, living life. You would never know or suspect what we are about to talk about based on outward appearances unless you are already living with these problems.

Let's start with a basic activity we do every day and sometimes multiple times a day: getting dressed.

Imagine not being able to dress yourself. We take this basic daily event for granted, and not a second thought goes to it. We just wake up and at some point put our clothes on. Well, for many obese people, it isn't that easy.

The ability to get dressed is all attributed to basic body mechanics. Arms and legs are only so long, and our bodies are designed to freely bend over, reach, and move. It's obvious that at some point, the sheer volume of body fat will decrease a person's range of motion and structurally block the hand from being able to reach the foot. The thick fat layers at the abdomen and thighs smashing up against each other leads to the inability to bend normally and with limited limb flexibility. Lower-body dressing is the first to go—socks, pants, shoes, and yes, even underwear. "What?" you might be asking. "You mean people are walking around underwearless?" Yeah, man, it's quite common. Many are also sockless, with slip-on shoes, sandals, or slippers. Take a look next time you're out and about. Why are so many obese people wearing sandals, flip-flops, or slippers . . . in the frickin' winter? Because most are physically not able to put on socks and tie shoes anymore.

You say, "The obese and morbidly obese people I encounter in public are not able to get dressed?" Well, there is a workaround to this dressing dilemma. Adaptive equipment can increase a person's ability to reach their lower body. You know, those long-handled sticks with a trigger at one end and a claw at the other, usually referred to as a "reacher" or a "grabber." A person can use one of those or a dressing stick to claw the waistband of underwear and pants, then with the increased length or reach provided by the stick, thread the garments over the feet and pull them up to a point where the other hand can finally physically grasp the waistband (usually at knee level) and yank it the rest of the way up. Socks can be slipped on with a tool called a sock aid, a three-fingered foldable device on two long ropes that allows you to stuff a sock on to it, flip it down to your feet, and with the two ropes yank the sock on over your foot. What about shoes? Well, laces are difficult to tie with a stick. You can add elastic laces and pretie them, but this is time consuming, so most obese people just wear slip-on shoes, flip-flops, or sandals.

This sounds like a lot of work, huh? Most obese patients I work with wear slip-on shoes and loose, baggy clothing. So loose they can whip the waistband down and thread it over their feet. Many just wear a single-piece nightgown or muumuu—and not because it's the new cool style! This dressing style is out of necessity. All that extra mass is a structural blockade between the upper body and the lower body. When it comes down to it, many obese people get their spouses, significant others, or kids to help them get dressed and avoid using adaptive equipment altogether because it's easier just to let someone else do it.

This mind-blowing knowledge must be enough to thrust your motivation train into high gear. I bet you're standing up, doing jumping jacks, or performing some other exercise right now. Right? No. Not yet. You're not feeling it. You don't care that much about getting yourself dressed or what clothing you wear. But maybe you're a bit provoked or intrigued? Okay, well, let's keep the momentum going. Let's keep that motivation train running and add fuel to the fire. We haven't even gotten into bathing yet!

"Oh, no! Not bathing. Please tell me differently," you're saying to yourself. Well, sorry—there is a reason BO (body odor) is common among people with a lot of extra body fat. For one, there is much more square footage of excretion tissue (how the skin releases oils, sweat, and toxins), and if the skin is rolling or folding up on itself, then things in the darkness cannot breathe. This sounds like a line in a horror movie. Well, take a sniff of fresh BO, and you'll feel like you're the superstar smack dab in the middle of a horror movie yourself.

It is difficult to reach all areas of skin on the body when, just like with dressing the arms, a layer of spongiform fat blocks you from reaching areas that are farther away, like your feet, back, or butt crack. Now, there are workarounds for this too. Just like using a reacher, sock aide, and long-handled shoe horn to aide in lower-body dressing, there are also tools for bathing. The adaptive equipment available for bathing is just as clever—like a long-handled bath brush and handheld shower head. Or there's getting another person to wash the hard-to-reach areas in the darkness for you. "Thanks for saving the best for me, Bob!" says Bob's wife as she washes his out-of-reach body parts. Now that's stoking the fire for you, right?

We have already listed many of the negative health effects of obesity, like increased risk of stroke, diabetes, and death. These detriments are well publicized by our government and schools, yet people still continue to grow larger and move less.

So again, we are turning this up a notch and openly revealing the unknown, secret, personal, and behind-the-scenes reality of obesity and morbid obesity when it comes to a person's quality of life. These topics are not openly talked about or publicized because we are worried about hurting people's feelings, rubbing people the wrong way, or being politically incorrect. Well, how the hell can we fix or heal a problem as big as the current obesity epidemic if we can't even talk about it?

On that note, let's blow the lid off this party can. Let's talk about what's in my opinion, based on my clinical observations and experiences treating thousands of patients over the years in the hospital setting, the worst and most life-altering impairment to self-care that obesity can cause.

The inability to wipe your own ass.

"What the hell! You didn't just go there." Yes, I did.' Cause it's super common. In fact, it's much more common a predicament than anyone realizes. And it's disturbing.

I work with lots of people every day who cannot wipe their own butt. In fact, I would guess that seven out of ten patients who have been admitted to a hospital and *ordered* by their doctors to work with therapists are overweight, obese, or morbidly obese.

Doctors do not order us to see healthy thin, muscular, or skinny people unless they've had surgery or have an unpreventable issue, or if they've ruined their bodies with smoking, drugs, alcohol, or an accident leading to trauma. The low percentage of leaner, lower-weight, active, and healthy people admitted to the hospital are usually there for natural reasons, like baby delivery, broken bones, or some other unpreventable issue.

Basically, healthy people don't need hospitals.

Unhealthy obese patients cannot wipe or poorly wipe after a bowel movement (BM), making a big mess of things due to poor reach ability. They are also eating a lot of greasy, unhealthy food and have multiple BMs a day. Hello, massive, stinky, much-too-frequent, explosive blow-outs.

"Well, how does it get wiped?" you're thinking.

The answer is already there in your mind; you're just blocking it from revealing itself openly because it is so unfathomable, and it's somewhat traumatic for the *non-healthcare worker*:

Another person wipes it.

. . . Or it doesn't get wiped.

This predicament is very sad and much too prevalent in the world. The inability to wipe your own ass after taking a dump is embarrassing and degrading, and it's a complete loss of all dignity or modesty for most people.

The other day I interviewed a gal at a spa in reference to Brazilian bikini waxing for obese clients. "Do you turn people away?" I asked. She replied with a sigh of disgust, "Oh, yeah, you wouldn't believe the stuff we see. We have to tell those people to go home and take care of that first." She was referring to the dirty state of a morbidly obese person's crotch and anus area that gets waxed. In healthcare, this is referred to as the peroneal or peri-area.

There are creative methods for cleaning the peri-area at home that cannot be replicated by an obese person once they have been taken out of their home and placed into a hospital.

Riding a beach towel is a common technique. With one arm grasping the towel in front and the other arm at the back, the person pulls or drags the towel back and forth through the anal-groin area until the crack is clean. Another technique is laying a towel on the edge of the bed or on the towel rack, then rubbing the booty up and down and all around until it is sufficiently cleaned, or as clean as can be expected in this situation. The poopy towel goes in the laundry, or sometimes multiple poopy towels a day if you're a frequent shitter or have diarrhea.

There are many other alternative methods to wipe your butt if you cannot reach it. One option is using a toilet aid. A toilet aid is a long-handled, usually curved, soft plastic and rubber contraption with a catch at the end to wrap toilet paper on. It will extend a person's reach to wipe that booty. Some toilet aids come with a carry case if you're traveling or out on the town. I mean, think about it. If you cannot wipe your butt without your toilet aid, then you definitely don't want to get stuck on a public toilet without it. If there is no beach towel available or sharable wall-mount toilet aid, then you are left with nothing other than pulling up those pants and hoping it doesn't leak through before you make it back home.

Don't worry, if you are obese and this hasn't motivated you enough to start eating restrictively and start an exercise program, there are cool new smart toilets. Smart toilets are high technology. Sitting down initiates a heated seat. After you've pinched off a loaf, the smart toilet will spray a warm-water wash at your butt crack until it is clean as a whistle. To finalize this grand toileting experience, the smart toilet will warm-air blow-dry your buttocks to its splendor.

Not all obese persons are stuck in this exact dilemma, but with different variations, they struggle to wipe that booty. It may not be as easy as when they were thinner, yet if they remain pretty flexible, likely those who are younger than older, they can get the job done using momentum and such.

The poopy-butt dilemma seems to predominantly affect the obese and morbidly obese who are sedentary and deconditioned, retiring, aging, getting sick more often, suffering from urinary tract infections and hygiene-related infections like cellulitis, or starting to need surgeries. They just cannot use flexibility, strength, or momentum to their advantage anymore.

Motivated yet? Well, you should be because this shit is real, and the older you get, the harder it is to backtrack.

EXERLEAN's Butt-Scale and Wipeability Meter was designed to help those visual learners out there. I've developed these simple visual parameters to measure wipeability. There are two basic factors involved in the ability to get a quality reach and wipe. One is the *length of the wiping arm* from shoulder to hand. This length can never change. You cannot separate your shoulder from the body, and your range of motion at the shoulder, elbow, wrist, and hands are fixed and have their limits. The second factor is *butt-cheek size and the open space/width of the butt crack*. The leaner or thinner a person is, the narrower the total butt width from outer hip edge to outer hip edge and the wider, more open the crack or space between the butt cheeks. The lean person with space between their butt cheeks is known as the clean shitter. The poop does not rub on the butt cheeks on the way out, leaving no trace of residue. The fatter the butt, the less open or tighter the butt crack and the wider the butt from outer hip edge to outer hip edge. In other words, the more obese the person, the less space between the cheeks until there is no space at all, like two balloons smashing together and drowning out the butt crack altogether. This is known as the dirty shitter. Poop smears on the cheeks on the way out, leaving much residue for cleanup, which requires more toilet paper, baby wipes, and work.

To get a visual of this scale, imagine sitting on a copy machine and taking a copy of your butt. The more obese the person, the wider the butt printout and also the narrower the butt crack.

EXERLEAN: Resolution for the physique transformation of a lifetime.

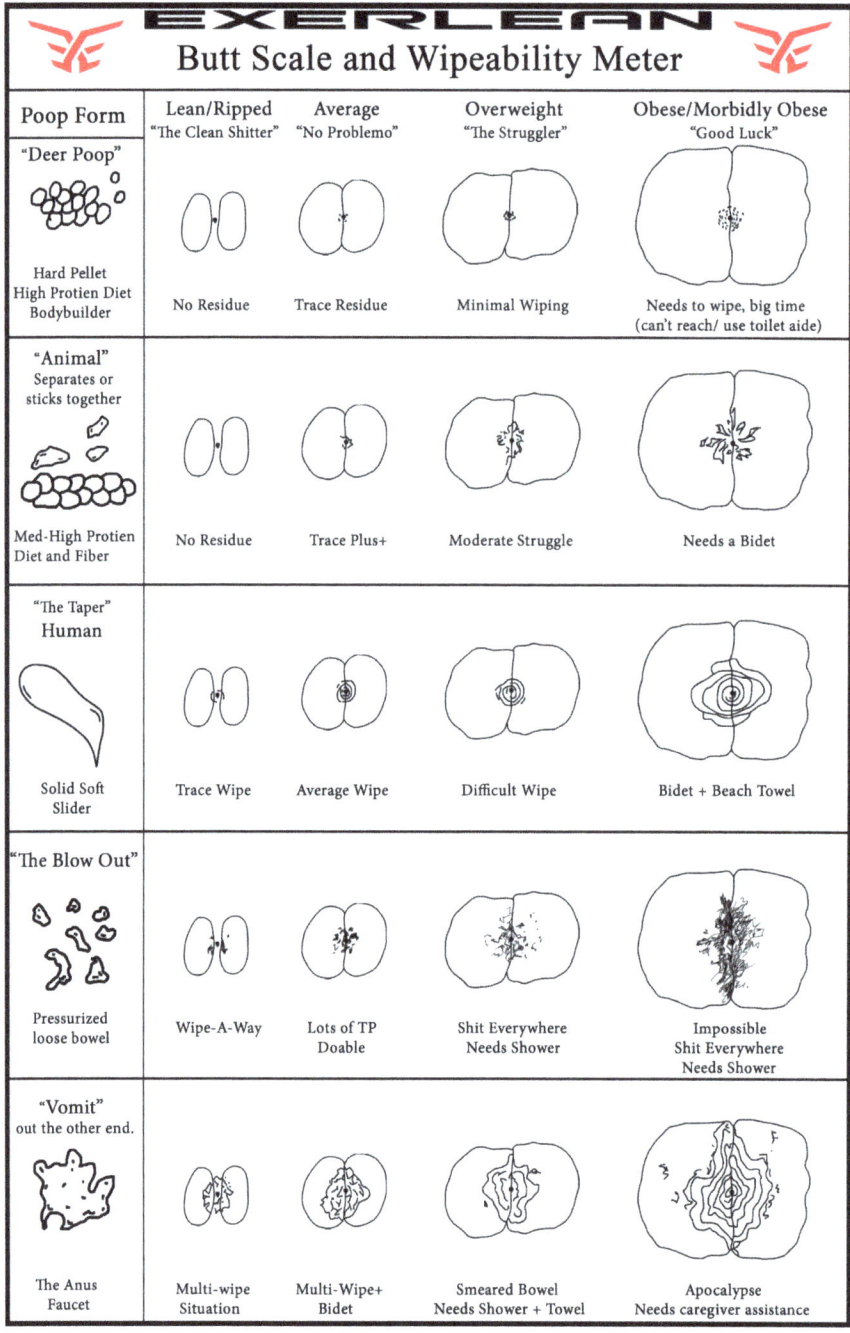

Chapter 4: Wipe Your Own!

EXERLEAN
Reachability Meter

"As the body widens, the shoulder to hand length remains the same. The further the hand gets from the buttocks, the harder...if not impossible it is to wipe."

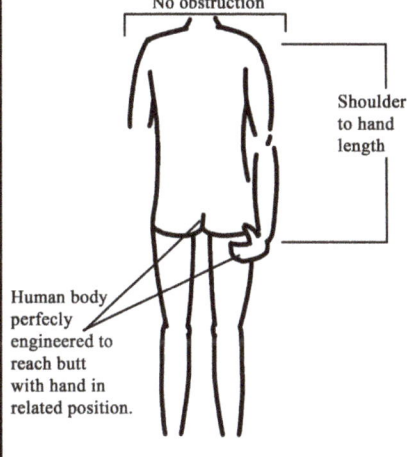

No obstruction
Shoulder to hand length
Human body perfecly engineered to reach butt with hand in related position.

Lean / Thin / Light

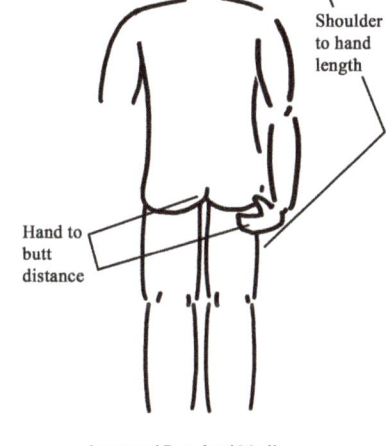

Shoulder to hand length
Hand to butt distance

Average / Regular / Medium

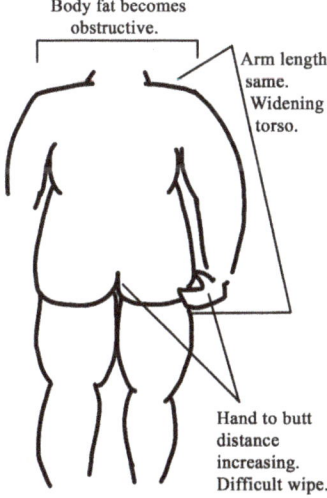

Body fat becomes obstructive.
Arm length same. Widening torso.
Hand to butt distance increasing. Difficult wipe.

Overweight / Plump / Moderately Heavy

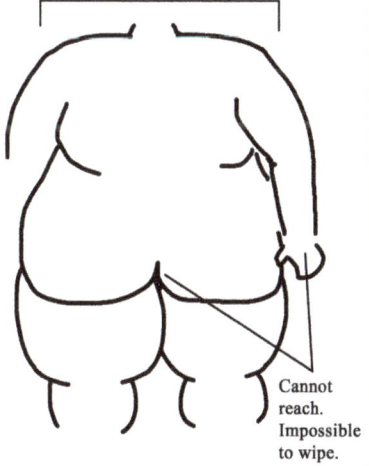

Width of torso and buttocks decreases reachability
Cannot reach. Impossible to wipe.

Obese / Morbidly Obese / Super Heavy

Adaptive methods and equipment can help a person wipe when they cannot reach the poop. For example, a toilet aide, an over-tiolet bidet, or smart toilet. The best remedy is to lose weight.

EXERLEAN 29

Now is your time to act. Remember! The current way of thinking, and the trends and statistics we have reviewed so far, are bad and in a sharp upward climb to oblivion.

The Obesiboomer generation is paying a high price and will continue to pay more physically, mentally, financially, and with decreased overall quality of life. As the prevalence of obesity continues to rise, so will the Obesiboomers' decline in occupational performance, community mobility, and self-care.

The well-publicized health detriments listed by the CDC, the World Health Organization (WHO), and the NIH will continue to skyrocket out of control.

The current education system in schools, in public health sectors, and on social media about the negative effects of obesity and how to deal with them is *obviously* not working!

In fact, the current social and education environment is teaching us that in a way, obesity is a "good thing" and should be accepted. Social media outlets and news broadcasts have been force-feeding us information and reeducation, brainwashing us into believing that being overweight, obese, and morbidly obese is beautiful, normal, and to be considered such.

Hate to break it to you—this is a nontruth.

A lie.

This kind of media and force-fed education is teaching our youth, average adults, and the general public that being overweight, obese, and morbidly obese should be considered normal and to accept it as such... . Bullshit!

Don't succumb to this ruse.

No wonder the obesity epidemic is afflicting so many youth, adults, and the elderly at rates exponentially increasing as every year passes. No wonder we as a species are becoming fatter and fatter year by year.

We need to change our way of thinking and our view on being overweight, obese, and morbidly obese.

We need to stay focused on the truth. The truth that excess body fat is a predictor of negative health consequences, and the more obese a person is, the worse the afflictions they will face, leading all the way to and possibly causing death.

This is the primary driver for me writing this book. I see what is happening in the hospitals, in schools, and in public, and I monitor the statistics on obesity. Nothing out there is working to halt the rising statistics on child, adult, and elderly obesity, and death is on the horizon. Nothing the government, schools, and medical community are doing is decreasing the rise in the obesity epidemic.

That is why I am approaching this problem at such a different angle.

I want to make a positive difference in people's lives and bring about a trend that will hopefully end the obesity epidemic—otherwise referred to as the Obesiboomer epidemic or pandemic, you might say. My goal is to give you enough ammunition. Enough reason to treat and prevent obesity now and for the rest of your life.

The Obesiboomer epidemic is spreading like wildfire, and the knowledge of health detriments like diabetes, stroke, heart attack, and death do not seem to be giving people enough ammunition or motivation to do the work, to make positive changes toward their health.

Hopefully, getting a glimpse into how being overweight, obese, or morbidly obese can affect the unseen, intimate, private, and very personal aspects of your life is enough knowledge, enough fuel, to explode that motivation train into full steam ahead. The negative side effects and reality of obesity we discuss openly in this book are meant to slap you across the face to get your attention, then reach inside you, grab your soul, and shake it around a bit. The goal is to help you retain this knowledge with the hope that it sticks in the back of your mind forever. You may not be ready to do something about your body fat now, but maybe down the road something from this book will click, and EXERLEAN will be waiting. I want you to think about all the devastating effects of obesity every time you are about to sink your teeth into something to eat. When you are eating, I want you to think about what specifically you are eating and whether it is necessary energy, whether it is healthy, and whether it will go toward healing your body or get sent straight to your ass to get stored there!

That, I hope, will help motivate you to do what is necessary now and for the rest of your life. To lose all the excess body fat and start exercising.

This is EXERLEAN: restrictive + healthy + balanced nutrition, daily exercise, and hyperactive activities of daily living. It's the formula for achieving happiness, longevity, and living without difficulty.

Daily exercise plus healthy and restrictive nutrition . . . you cannot have one without the other.

you + EXERLEAN = maximal health

EXERcising daily + eating LEAN
EXER + LEAN = EXERLEAN

If all Obesiboomers follow and live by the EXERLEAN formula, there will eventually be no more Obesiboomers. The perfect scenario would be a shift of the obesity statistics in a different direction. A new era of humanity focused on their health management, working toward maintaining a healthy body weight and staying active with work, play, and exercise. Maybe this book will help create an army of health nuts, fitness gurus, health and wellness coaches, bodybuilders, CrossFitters, powerlifters, gymnasts, dancers, martial artists, runners, bicyclers, hikers, and other physically active people. The dawn of the Leanbodiboomers.

You're reading this book because you want change. You want to do something different from the norm. Something that will help you down the path to looking better, feeling better, having more energy, being stronger, sleeping better, elevating your sex and libido, and living a longer and rewarding healthstyle.

Good! That is why I wrote this book, and trust me, it will help you make radical changes to the way you look at life, yourself, and the human body, and how to remediate and/or prevent the health detriments of obesity in your life.

Please don't skip ahead.

The information in the book from beginning to end is strategically laid out to help you transform yourself into the *best you ever*. I want you to fully grasp why this works and why you are doing what you are going to be doing. This information will help you for the rest of your life. Learn the rules, principles, and process, then you can achieve a life living lean forever. Some of the materials are designed with the intent to provoke you, to wake up your inner passion, and to help reboot your healthstyle, which will help you achieve a *real* transformation.

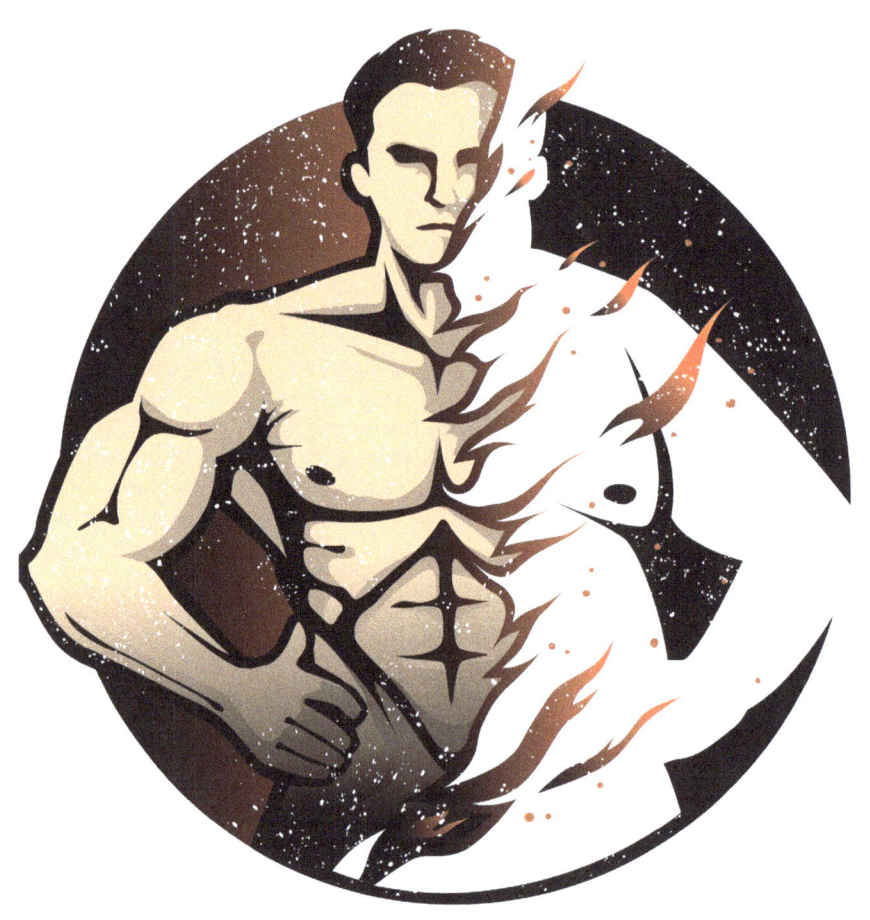

CHAPTER 5
Dadbodinator

Now that we have beat the crap out of the negative effects of obesity and have instilled in ourselves an obvious need to start obliterating body fat and initiate an exercise program of some sort, what's next? When it comes to the point where a person decides it is time to lose body fat and start an exercise program, where and when should they start? It seems a common thread to start a new dieting and weight loss program with a New Year's resolution. Many employers offer incentives to enroll and engage in personal health and wellness or a program to follow during the new year. This is a good way to start your healthstyle change but only if the new year is right around the corner. Otherwise, the time to start is now. Do not procrastinate. Your life depends on it.

If you already have knowledge of and experience on how to turn your body into a fat incinerator and how to launch a fitness and weight training program, then kudos to you. Hopefully some of the nutrition and exercise ideas presented in the EXERLEAN program will help make your journey more interesting.

Most people, however, do not know what exercise is or what to eat. We learn some basic health knowledge in elementary school, middle school, and high school, but not enough.

In my elementary to high school experience, there was very little if any education on how to eat for weight management and longevity, how to promote fat burning, and the art of bodybuilding, and very brief education and training on weights and exercise.

Nowadays, school systems' fitness programs are much different from gym classes of yesteryear. Many schools have made PE an elective. Gym teachers do their best to educate youth on how to take care of their bodies but within the policies, restrictions, guidelines, and rules of their governing school systems. This approach may work for some kids, but it is definitely not working for most, otherwise the youth obesity rate would stop climbing exponentially.

There is a gap in or deletion of the necessary jargon and knowledge youth need to empower themselves to prioritize their health now and for the rest of their lives. Word usage and tone are key in provoking a lasting response when it comes to eating and activity. The absolute truth is necessary to make an educated decision about anything in life. Yet the education system is delivering an unmemorable message to our youth because it does not allow teachers to use provoking language or speak negatively about obesity and drill home its negative effects because they are so concerned about hurting someone's feelings or being politically incorrect. Their hands are tied behind their backs. Can you blame the school systems, though? We already acknowledged the fear the media and social networks have instilled in us about being offensive or discriminating when it comes to weight. This bullshit environment has led to a lackluster, low emotional response in youth about being fat—many don't even care. Consequently, teachers aren't able to teach in a way that will trigger change in eating and exercise habits.

Given these circumstances, it's no surprise that when kids become adults, they lack the necessary knowledge, desire, or power to actually make a difference in their lives by making disciplined eating and exercising decisions. People do not know how to live out and adopt healthy behaviors and habits. Therefore, everyone from youth to adult needs to seek out a new method and acquire knowledge on their own. The best way to acquire the necessary knowledge to change one's self for the better is through books on sports nutrition, fitness, and bodybuilding and through coaching from proven expert trainers.

These people have experience and expertise in their own lives and walk the talk.

Does the creator or author of the weight loss program, diet protocol, or book you're interested in or thinking about undertaking walk the talk, or are they obese? If they don't lead by example, then you should question the validity of the content. Think about it—how can the author, creator, TV host, or whoever help you get lean if they are not lean themselves? If a person has never been lean and ripped, how can they possibly educate from the context of factual personal experience and knowledge? If an "expert" doesn't have proof of concept, they likely are just regurgitating information from other resources that may or may not work. This is why you should not hire an obese personal trainer or nutrition guru. They cannot help you . . . not for the long term.

You need the truth. You need to be guided by example. You need to follow the path of least resistance to achieve maximal fat loss and at the same time adopt a worthwhile and rewarding exercise regimen. I would like to offer my services. That is why I wrote this book. I dream of and hope to provoke a response in you. I hope that the words in this book light a fire inside that will propel you toward making positive changes in your life. I aim to help you fill in the gaps. The gaps that were left empty at some point in your education thus far. We, you and I, are going to fill those gaps with tools and knowledge that will unshackle your body fat incinerator. Yup, you have an internal body fat incinerator, or furnace, you might say. It is called your metabolism. You just need to learn how to ignite it, fuel it with body fat, and then crank up the thermostat.

Maybe you are pissed off for reading this book and will walk away no different. I hope not. Regardless, I believe the information you have read thus far will stick with you if you've read up to this point. Even if you fail to make a stand now, you will at least have this information lingering in your mind forever. The EXERLEAN introduction, statistics, statements, and facts will be dancing around in the back of your mind, and someday off in the future, you will hopefully decide to take a stand against the devastating and deadly status of obesity. EXERLEAN will be waiting.

From this point forward, I would like to be your trainer. Your trainer for life. I am writing this book to trigger a response from you, to help you make lifelong habit and behavior changes. This book will be around forever, and I will not. The knowledge and tools provided here will be available to anyone who needs them for as long as books exist.

If the twenty-one years it took me to finally finish this book makes a positive difference and changes just one person's life, then all the work I've put toward developing this book were totally worth it. I ultimately hope that this book does more than that, though. I aim to spark a flame in the masses and move the statistics on the worldwide obesity epidemic in a declining direction. I aim to tip the scales. I hope this book triggers other writers, fitness experts, nutritional coaches, and the media to speak real about obesity and use truth to motivate change. I want people to question everything they have been taught, think is truth, and believe is healthy.

When you decide to take the plunge, hiring a personal trainer is a great idea, especially when it comes to navigating the gym and using unfamiliar exercise equipment. I recommend finding a trainer who actually is or has been ripped and has the right knowledge to share with you. Nobody knows how to harness the power of thermogenesis (incinerating body fat) better than a seasoned competitive bodybuilder or former bodybuilder. Not a wannabe bodybuilder, or a bodybuilder in the making, but a proven competitive bodybuilder with years of experience battling it out on stage. Ask for pictures to prove their success in obtaining a super-lean physique and helping clients achieve the same. Better yet, choose a bodybuilder who also has an education in the sciences of the human body.

It is important to pay attention to who you're taking advice from. Do they have enough experience? Do they have expert credentials? Do they have expert knowledge on the human body and its physiology? Are you taking advice or paying someone who may only have some gym rat or sports experience, has heart but lacks experience, is motivated but without expertise, and who works at a pizza parlor part time and has read a few books on fitness? Just because someone is a therapist or an MD or has PhD does not automatically make them an expert in the field of getting lean. But if that educated expert is not only smart and educated but also lives lean, competes lean, and can teach lean, that's your trainer!

Not everyone can afford to hire a personal trainer. It is worth it, but it's expensive. It can range anywhere from $35 to $125 an hour, depending on the trainer.

For the price of a book, I will be your trainer. I've written this book and more to be your guide. I have YouTube, Instagram, Facebook, Tumbler, and other networking channels with free videos to help inspire and educate people with meal prep, exercise, and other lean life hacks. EXERLEAN has a website (www.exerlean.com) to continue the knowledge train.

Think about it. Hiring a personal trainer for one hour will cost you at least forty bucks, or you can buy this book and many more for much less and be able to refer over and over again to them for as long as necessary. In my mind, this book and many like it are much undervalued.

I am a licensed and nationally registered occupational therapist. I have decades of experience in outpatient cardiopulmonary rehabilitation and inpatient acute care. I am a Certified Aging-in-Place Specialist (CAPS). I have been a National Physique Committee (NPC) competitive bodybuilder since 1997 and have been absolutely shredded many times over. I am a certified fitness trainer (CFT) and have helped many clients earn better bodies. I am a former competitive powerlifter with experience in competition weightlifting. I have ACLS and BLS certifications (advanced cardiac life support and basic life support). I was the Gold's Gym poster boy in 1997. I placed top forty in the nation competing in the MaxFormation 2000 and was in the *Ripley's Believe It or Not* feature on Kelly Nelson, at the time the world's oldest female competitive bodybuilder.

I know this stuff left to right, up, down, and all around. The physique transformation arena is like breathing for me, it's automatic.

Well, on that note, I have got a confession. I formerly worked as the dough master at a pizza parlor! When I was nineteen years old, I would open up the hut at 6:00 a.m., mix up all the dough, set it out to rise, then get all the toppings ready for the lunch buffet. I loved that job! It was fun and I'm the early morning type. After the hut I would go to my second job at Waste Management, washing trucks until 10:00 p.m. I had a third job on the weekends working at Kentucky Fried Chicken. Eventually my job as a truck washer was upgraded to garbageman.

I do have my early days of being a gym rat for sure. While a garbageman and competition bodybuilder on the side, I wrote my first book called *The Garbageman's Diet*. I wrote the book to help my coworkers at the time get in better shape. I became a certified personal trainer and worked at Gold's Gym while working full time as a garbageman and attending college at night with almost a double credit load. I wanted to complete all my prerequisites so I could apply to graduate school.

I was accepted to the OT school at Eastern Washington University, quit my garbageman job, and that fall started OT school. While in school, I won first place and best poser trophies in my twelfth NPC bodybuilding competition. I continued to work as a personal trainer as often as I could on the weekends and college breaks. Another side job I fit in was working as an exercise specialist in outpatient cardiopulmonary rehab.

OT school was the single most difficult, stressful, and challenging period of my life, but I won the battle and earned my degree. I immediately received a full-time job in an acute care hospital as an OT. I'm telling you all this information to reassure you that you're currently following the path of a well-educated, experienced, and credible trainer who walks the talk.

But I'm far from perfect. I have had my own personal experience with eating poorly and not exercising. I've fallen off track, gained body fat and become overweight, lost muscle mass and strength, become sedentary, and succumbed to an unhealthy version of me. Hence the birth of the Dadbodinator—me. Here's how the Dadbodinator was born.

Starting back in 1998, I was the trainer at Gold's Gym who would always preach to people that there were no excuses to eat poorly and not exercise. This is true, but we as human beings develop habits or rituals very quickly, good ones and bad ones.

In my first year out of college, 2004, I entered and won another bodybuilding competition. I was enjoying my new career as an OT. I met the girl of my dreams and got married.

Like many . . . this is where I began to lose my way.

Over the next year, I ate worse and worse and made it to the gym less and less. Eating high-calorie, fat-laden meals and eating out with my new relatives slowly became the norm. As I was and still am addicted to spending time with my wife, I slowly lost focus on my health and worked out sporadically and without passion. Within a couple of years, I quit going to the gym altogether. Once my son was born, it was over. With working full time, making time for my family, and juggling all my side jobs, I was left with no time to go to the gym.

Excuses.

I never felt okay with this. I knew the consequences of an inactive, unhealthy life, and I was a competitive bodybuilder at heart who sought health and wellness and yearned to throw weights around at the gym.

We all have excuses. Work and family were mine. I spent the next ten years of my life, 2007 to 2017, working as a therapist and helping others get stronger. I had been working for years promoting an active life of health and wellness and all the while infrequently investing in my own body.

The first five years of my dadbod—the body of a man after getting married and having kids, eating like crap, and not working out—life was not bad. The effects of all my previous years of dedicated training and muscle memory helped me stay strong and in relatively decent shape. But the next five to ten years is where everything started falling apart, literally. I started losing my muscle mass, gaining body fat, and losing strength, which led to me getting injured at work. Being a therapist or a nurse in a hospital can be dangerous due to the demanding physical loads when lifting patients out of bed and then helping them stand up and mobilize to a chair, wheelchair, or toilet. Have you ever tried to move a person who cannot move themselves?

It's vital to be in top physical condition in a job like this to prevent physical injury. Well, "top physical condition," that I was not in. I was conditioned for injury and started getting injuries and muscle strains way too easily and much too often. My out-of-shape dadbod also led to constant back pain and intermittent bouts of foot, knee, wrist, and neck pain depending on how the workweek went.

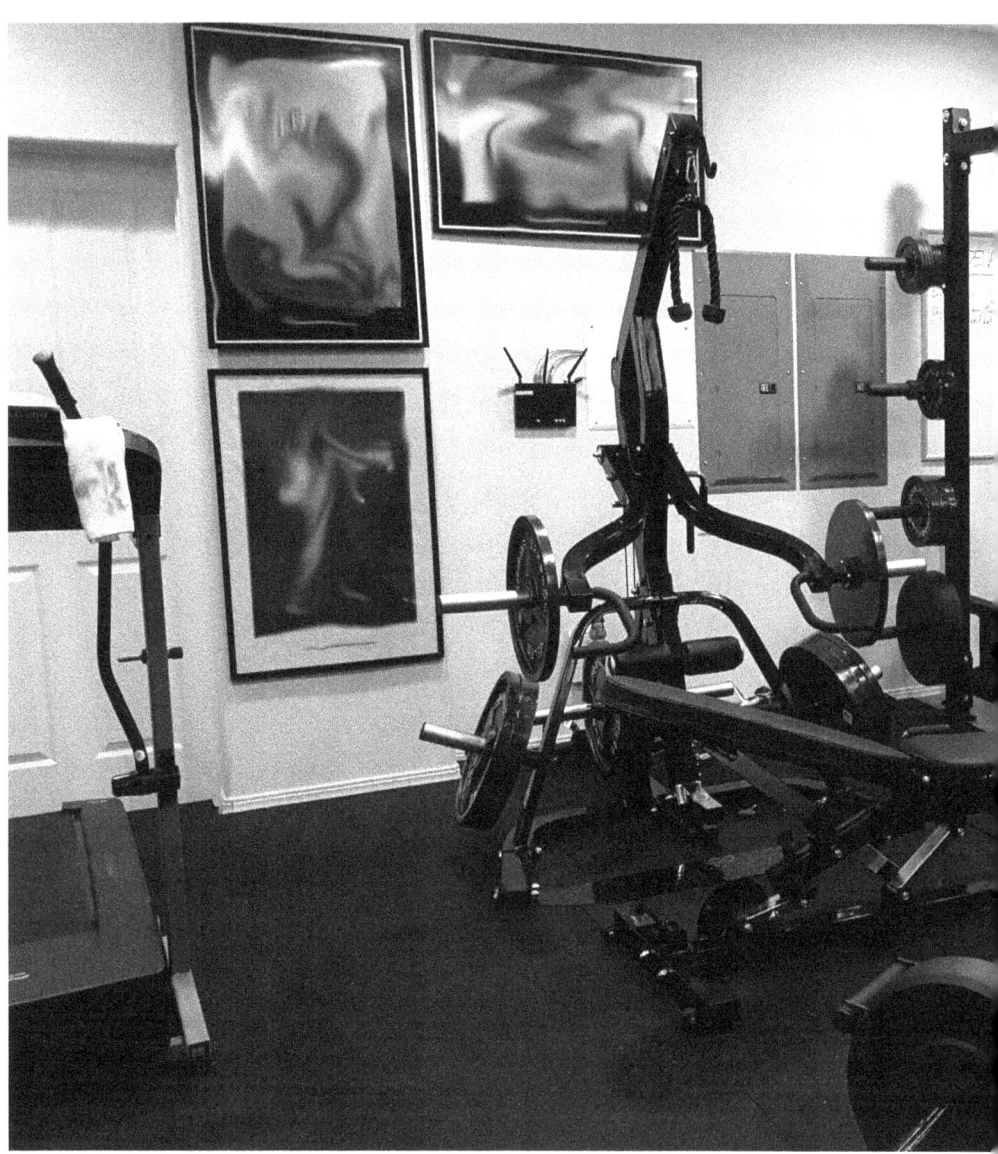

1: Rogue Power Rack
2: Powertec Levergym
3: Operator Barbell
4: Bumper Plates
5: Olympic Weights
6: Dumbells
7: Adjustable Bench
8: Bands

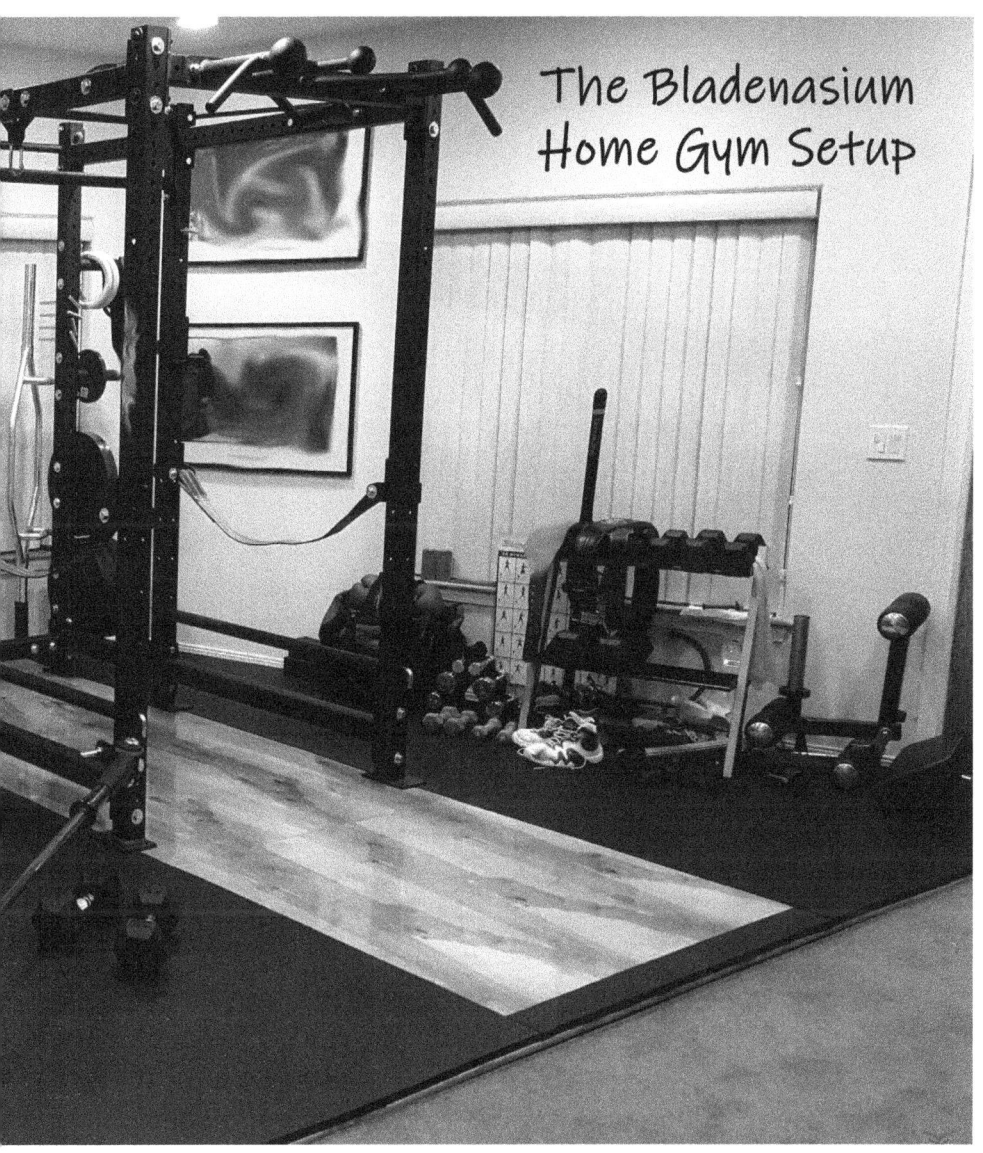

9: Horse stall matts/3/4 inch rubber flooring
10: Deadlift and Squat Platform
11: Arnold Schwarzenegger Posters
12: Bodybuilding Trophies (not shown)
13: Accessory grips, handles, ropes, attachments, and collars.
14: Treadmill and Precorn Elyptical (not shown)
15: Landmine and Tbar row handle
16: A whole lot of fun planning and putting this setup together

Over time the constant pain, increasing fatigue, and generalized weakness took its full toll. I started becoming stressed, depressed, and desperate to find a way out of my unhealthy and unsustainable predicament. I knew if I didn't change the situation for the long term, I could someday end up disabled, unable to keep up with the physical demands of my job, and with a future less fulfilling. As we age it only gets more difficult to change, and if we are not living a healthy, restrictive, and balanced life, the retirement years can be spent dealing with constant health issues.

I don't know exactly when or why, but I finally snapped and decided to take a stand. I made a conscious and vivid statement to myself: "Time to end this shit! Time to do the work! Time to change my ways! Time to get in the best shape of my life and keep it forever! Time to get strong again. Time to become conditioned for the demands of my job. Time to feed my body with food it needs and avoid the foods it doesn't. Time to burn off all the excess body fat."

"Let's do this!" became my mantra for the journey ahead.

I spent weeks brainstorming ideas, schedules, finances, time, family, work, and more trying to come up with a plan that would not fail. Failure was not an option. I had to make sure nothing would derail me on my path to reach my goals.

A major problem I needed to solve—and also the main contributor to my failure to make it to the gym the last ten years—was lack of *time*. I was so busy with work, taking care of the kids and all their school functions, and other stuff. Packing a gym bag, loading it in the car, and actually going to and working out at a gym was going to be so inconvenient that I knew it might ultimately lead to failure.

I figured out that if I had a home gym, a place where I could hit the weights, exercise, and perform other conditioning activities at my convenience, then my family could access me as needed. I could simply help them in between sets or exercises. If I had a home gym, I could schedule my workout or just do it on a whim.

I realized the benefits of having a home gym would be crucial in meeting my goals. So I sat down with my wife and laid out my proposal.

"Sweetie, I need to change things. I'm tired of getting hurt at work and of being weak, fat, and feeling like crap."

"I've made a commitment to myself to take massive action and to do something about it."

"Weight training and exercise are vital tools to help me reach my goals."

"I have limited time after work to get in a good workout and still get all my husband and dad jobs completed."

"I've researched gym equipment, and there is a lot more available nowadays than when I was younger. There are power racks, multigyms, systems, benches, and accessories that allow for most powerlifting, bodybuilding, and cross-training workouts."

"If we have a home gym with all the necessary equipment for me to do the basic lifts like squats, bench presses, and deadlifts, then I can work out in the convenience of our own home and at any time."

"Instead of investing in a gym membership, we can invest in building a home gym that will be there forever and whenever we need to hit it. The kids can learn to use it too!"

"What do you think?"

"Do it!" she said. BOOM!

Thus began the designing process of our future home gym. We decided where to set it up and then made a list of the necessary startup equipment, knowing that over time we could keep adding to it.

Purchasing everything necessary to build the home gym of our choice was a small fortune, about the price of a new hot tub. Once we drafted the final order list, we decided to wait and execute our purchase plan on Black Friday to capture some sales and shipping deals.

In the meantime, I went to Home Depot and purchased four-by-eight-foot sheets of plywood for the gym flooring, then to the feed store for some four-by-eight-foot stall mats—the thick rubber flooring used in horse stalls . . . or commercial gyms. I designed the shape of the area for the gym floor or floor print, then began construction. I cut and laid out all the plywood in the shape of the gym floor design. Then I fastened the sheets of plywood together with decking plates and flush-head screws. Now we had a good visual of the area our gym floor would encompass.

The anticipation and excitement was starting to churn . . .

In the spot where we planned to set up the power rack, I installed, sanded, and epoxy-coated a twelve-by-four-foot sheet of finish-grade plywood for the deadlift and squatting platform. Next, I laid six four-by-eight-foot stall mats over the plywood gym floor, butted them up edge to edge, and then trimmed the edges with a box cutter.

Once the power rack platform and stall mats were all placed and trimmed, I fastened them down with flush-head screws—black for the stall mats and copper colored for the platform. Ahh, beautiful! I thought to myself. Now I could look at the floor plan and visualize myself exercising and getting in shape. What a wonderful feeling realizing this was all really happening. It was then time to fill up the gym with some exercise equipment.

I spent hours over the course of weeks researching gym equipment. On my list was a power rack, which would allow me to both squat and bench without a spotter. Power racks come with safeties that offer protection from dropping the weight on yourself. If you lose power during a lift and need to let the weight down, the safeties are right there to catch the weight at the bottom of the movement. Also, power racks have a multitude of available accessories and options to add to the plethora of exercise options. I planned on purchasing a few add-on accessories including a pull-up bar, a landmine attachment, pegs for banding attachments, a dip bar, and a ring and rope setup.

I also wanted a separate easy-to-use multigym. I looked at different models like the Bowflex, Nautilus, Precor, Weider, Marcy, and others. I ultimately decided on the Powertec LeverGym because it uses free weights instead of a weight stack or bands. The ability to use free weights was very important for me as I had a long history of powerlifting and using free weights for most of my exercise or workout regimen.

I compiled a well-thought-out and designed list of equipment and accessories to order and anxiously awaited the next three weeks for Black Friday to arrive.

On Black Friday I woke up at about 5:00 a.m. and went online to check for the best prices. I made my largest purchase of equipment and accessories through Rogue Fitness, taking advantage of free shipping as gym equipment and weights are heavy and therefore expensive to ship. My second order for the Powertec LeverGym was straight through the manufacturer's website.

I also added the leg and preacher curl accessories for the LeverGym.

My third and final order was through walmart.com for about 750 pounds of free weights and various other workout and exercise accessories.

BOOM! The buttons were clicked. The money was spent. My home gym, which I refer to as the Bladenasium, was almost complete. Now the wait.

There is something powerful about having a start date to a weight loss, workout, or body transformation program. It builds anticipation and excitement. It allows prep time to figure out a workout plan, go shopping for groceries, order nutritional supplements, and, in my case, build a home gym. A start date conjures anticipation for work and brews mental preparation. When the date finally arrives, the built-up motivation will carry us through the initial grueling, mentally challenging days to weeks of calorie restriction, workout fatigue, and muscle aching. This motivation train will help us persevere through the rough waters breaking deep-seated, unhealthy habits and replacing them with new active and healthy ones.

With my start date weeks ahead and my home gym somewhere in shipping, my motivation train was coming in fast and strong. My cupboards were stocked with whey protein powder, vitamins, antioxidants, omegas, and shaker jugs ready at the wait. Years and years of knowledge on burning body fat, building muscle, strengthening, training, and competition were ready to be put to work again.

The pre-workout and diet preparation phase is fun, exciting, and healthy. It is a process of self-discovery and acknowledgment of where you are at the time and where you want to be in the future. It is a period of confidence building, positive thinking, and self-actualization. In goal setting, we create an active plan in our minds. We create a map for the process and the work, and we visualize how we will feel along the way. This momentum-building process prepares you mentally and emotionally for the journey to come.

During this waiting period, you will catch up on current exercise trends, home gym possibilities, and commercial gym memberships, classes, and rates. You will learn about current and popular supplements, meal replacements, fasting formulas, and workout routines.

In the back of your mind, you can see that all this work is for you, improving you and helping you take care of your body.

It is all fantastic!

The current trend is to repeat this "pre-workout and diet preparation phase" after the holidays, after a vacation, or at the start of a new year. The majority of fad diets seem to support this concept.

Not anymore!

Not with EXERLEAN!

Remember this and say it to yourself over and over again:

"Enough of the never-ending cycle of yo-yo dieting and on-and-off workouts. No more losing weight then getting fat, losing weight then getting fat."

Here are some statements you can repeat out loud or in your head to help gain focus for your transformation:"I'm taking a stand!"

1. "I'm creating an active lifestyle that sticks."
2. "Eating healthy and restrictively is the best natural path I can take to prevent obesity and obesity-related diseases and disability in my life."
3. "Exercising and engaging in an active lifestyle coupled with restrictive, purposeful eating will give me the best chances at longevity and mental health."
4. "I am in control of myself and my choices."
5. "I choose to put all my heart and soul into this process."
6. "This process will help me lose body fat, get stronger, and feel healthy."
7. "I'm going to look better."
8. "I'm going to burn the fat."
9. "I'm going to be strong."
10. "I'm going to feel awesome!"
11. "I'm not going to let anyone stop or hinder me from achieving my goals."
12. "I'm going to do the work."
13. "Screw the naysayers!"
14. "I will wipe my own to the end of days!"

CHAPTER 6
Bodinomics: The Economy of the Human Body

Now that you know who I am, my story, and that I walk the talk, have expert credentials, a lifetime of experience, and the balls to say it how it is—that is, to speak the truth—you can sit back and learn, absorb, and prepare yourself for the journey ahead. I want to help you change your life for the better. To launch the next phase of your life.

Transformation

Up to this point, we have talked about the negative effects of obesity on self-care, community mobility, and quality of life. We have reviewed the negative effects obesity has on our body's physiology, leading to early onset diabetes, heart disease, stroke, a myriad of other diseases, ailments, disability, and ultimately death.

I believe none of us wants to live in a way less than what we've imagined or dreamed of. None of us grow up dreaming of becoming fat, diseased, disabled, or enduring poor quality of life. There should be no more argument or contemplation about obesity and its undesired status in modern-day society.

It is not too late for most of us, and change is a good thing, especially when it involves purposeful, positive, goal-oriented, and life-altering movement forward.

From this point on, we are going to move into the EXERLEAN program and its transformation protocols. Let's move on to the information that will change everything.

To be successful in anything, we must do the necessary research and gain the knowledge required to implement the goal, change something, and finish the project. You would not want to hire a plumber whose knowledge is limited to electricity and wiring, right? Of course not! You want a plumber who has knowledge of pipes and drains. The same goes with the process of losing all that body fat. You are the person who will be doing all the work and tackling the job at hand. Only you can control what you eat, what you do, and how you feel. So just like the plumber needs to have knowledge of pipes and drains, you need to have knowledge of nutrition, exercise, and how to harness the power of thermogenesis, or fat burning.

First, we are going to lay out the foundation of basic information that is necessary for you to understand why you're doing what you're doing and what you are about to experience.

The Cost-Benefit Analysis

In economics, there is a simple decision-making approach called the cost-benefit analysis (CBA). For every choice or decision we make, there will be one of two possible outcomes: choose it or don't choose it, yes or no, go or stop. Each choice has two attributes we must weigh when making a decision—a cost or price paid, and a benefit or reward. For example, if I want to buy a new truck, two paradigms exist. The first is the cost of the truck. To determine this, I must write down the costs: the actual money spent on the vehicle, the debt acquired with interest, the stress of the debt, less money in the budget every month, and the expected costs of gas, parking, storage, vehicle expenses, and repairs. The second are the benefits, which I also must write down for analysis: comfort, luxury, safety, transportation, the ability to work, a nice stereo, and happiness. With the two lists of the costs and the benefits, we can compare and make a decision.

Chapter 6: Bodinomics: The Economy of the Human Body

Cost-Benefit Analysis: Buy a New Truck?

Costs	Benefits
$50,000	Can pull a trailer
Excessive fuel	Comfortable seats
Expensive repairs	Transportation to work and within community
Insurance, tags, registration	Four-wheel drive
Parking costs	Can use truck bed for hauling
	Seats the whole family
	Smells great and has a nice sounding stereo

    The cost-benefit analysis is objective. It is not entangled by emotion or confusion. The outcome is based on a logical decision made by weighing the costs and the benefits, in which the decider must or should always choose the heavy-handed beneficial route. In the example of buying a truck, if the cost or negatives of buying the truck outweigh the benefits or positives, then without a thought the truck should not be purchased. And vice versa—if the benefits far outweigh the costs, then the choice should be to purchase the truck. The cost-benefit analysis ensures the least regret in a decision.

    Regret is something we should strive to avoid in all areas of our lives. This belief is shared by Jeff Bezos, owner of Amazon and the richest man in the world. Bezos chooses to minimize regret, or as he terms it, *regret minimization*. Less regret leads to more reward. In life, a choice should never be made unless the benefits outweigh the costs, whether you're choosing a spouse, buying a boat, accepting a job, hiring an employee, deciding what to eat, deciding when to go left or right, or deciding to walk or drive. In a nonemotional and logical process, CBA will lead us forward in a positive direction. That is, only if we execute the heavy-handed beneficial choices and forgo the heavy-handed costly choices in life.

Cost-Benefit Analysis: Eat the Donut?

Costs	Benefits
Gain body fat	Instant gratification and reward
Hyperglycemia	Tastes great
Leads to diabetes	Energy boost
Insulin spike	
Adds to arteriosclerosis	
Energy crash	
… the costs outweigh the benefits. Do not eat the donut.	

One of the most important areas of life where CBA should be applied is our health. Bodinomics is an EXERLEAN set of CBA-based laws or principles dealing with the economy of the human body.

body + economics = Bodinomics

Bodinomics takes into consideration the physiology, science, behaviors, habits, self-care, work, play, and psychosocial aspects of humanity and helps us make the "beneficial" choices we need to make in order to move forward in a positive direction. If a person continues to make heavy-handed costly decisions about their body, then their life journey will be a progressively negative transformation until finally and very likely they experience an early death—the cost of their bad decisions.

And vice versa—if a person continues to make heavy-handed beneficial decisions about their body, their transformation or life journey will be progressively moving forward with positive momentum until finally and likely they experience the latest possible death—the benefit of a life filled with positive choices.

CHAPTER 7
Bodinomics: Fuel

D O NOT BLAME obesity or being overweight on food, fast-food joints, or the world. Obesity is a result of a decision: To eat or not to eat? Obesity is the product of overconsumption over time. Obesity is the benefit of a person's decisions when it comes to eating in excess and consistently choosing the heavy-handed negative food choices. When a person goes against the CBA and the laws` of Bodinomics and chooses the heavy-handed costly decision, the "benefit" becomes the negative result. In this case, obesity is the benefit of making cumulative heavy-handed costly decisions, and the cost of eating too much is the loss of attaining a lean, healthy body. In other words, your fat ass and cellulite is the reward for continually eating too much shit over time!

The benefit of overconsumption is to store body fat. The cost of overconsumption always far outweighs the benefit and should be avoided by any means necessary. But that is not what most people are doing, obviously, since greater than 70 percent of adults are overweight. Sadly, this statistic is only rising due to the overwhelming heavy-handed choice of overconsumption, which continues contributing to the obesity epidemic.

If you put too much fuel in the gas tank, it will overflow and spill out down the side of your car, right? This is also what happens with the human body. Too much food—or fuel—equals an overflow of food into body fat storage.

A car fuel tank has a fixed volume. You cannot put more in the tank than the tank can hold. Aside from that, the gas pump has an automatic shut-off mechanism to prevent the overflow of fuel.

The human body works in the same way. We have a "fixed" fuel system called our metabolism. At minimum, we need fuel for breathing and other basic functions. This is referred to as basal metabolic rate, or BMR. This is how much fuel, or *calories*, your body needs in a day just to stay alive—to pump the heart, circulate blood, breathe, and operate other autonomic body functions. Add work to the BMR, and this is referred to as your total daily energy expenditure (TDEE). If you add more fuel, or calories, then your TDEE will overflow straight into your ass.

Regardless of the size of your tank, there is no automatic shut-off mechanism at the pump.

You are the pump!

You control how much fuel goes in the tank.

You control or prevent overflow with your hand, fork, and mouth.

The physical tank that holds the fuel or calories in the human body is the stomach. The stomach does not correlate to BMR. In fact, if you stuff it full, the result will most likely be overflow and body fat storage. People who overeat have likely stretched their stomachs, creating a bigger void to fill, leading to even greater overflow and body fat storage.

Your stomach is not the problem. Your BMR is not the problem. The problem is you—the fuel pump—and putting too much fuel in the gas tank.

I've heard all the excuses in the world when it comes to overeating, and it's all bullshit. We dance around, avoid, and point fingers at everything except the simple truth: I put too much fuel in the tank, and now I'm stuck with the results . . . body fat.

This is science. There is no gray area. It's not your frickin' meds or your bad knee. It's not your mother's or your brother's bad choices, nor your doctor or your work. It's not the restaurant where you *chose* to dine or the influence of your friends.

The gray-area excuses go on and on like the erosion of the great Egyptian pyramids. None of these excuses give you any right or reason to stuff your face with whatever the hell you want and in any reckless quantity. If anything, most of the gray-area excuses, which sadly are real dilemmas, require less and even more restrictive and calculated eating than a typical active and healthy individual anyway.

Do not despair! You can change your way of thinking.

Bodinomics deals with the economy of the human body. The body has a complex economy or system dealing with ins and outs of fuel or vital nutrients, chemistry, hormones, organ function, circulation, respiration, digestion, and mental function. The human body strives to achieve a state of homeostasis, or balance, within its autonomic or automatic body systems, all organs, mental health, and physical environment. The choices we make regarding food chemistry and activity, including exercise, play a vital role in our homeostatic predicament. The rules, tools, and laws of Bodinomics can help you learn to achieve and maintain a healthy and well state of homeostasis in your body.

Now what? Knowing all this, what are you going to do? Nothing—no process, fad diet, FDA recommendation, Dr. Whoever diet, and the plethora of other media-driven programs aimed at weight loss—is halting the rise in the prevalence of obesity.

So . . . how about doing something different?

I mean, what the hell do we have to lose? If what is available is not working for the majority of the team, then it would be asinine and very inefficient to keep doing the same thing over and over again, achieving the same results every time.

Let's clarify what's happening. So far, today's health or weight loss plans have not stopped—and some have possibly contributed to—the rise in prevalence of obesity on a massive scale, from child to elder adult. So, maybe you should separate yourself from the lemmings.

The good news:

Obesity is treatable.

Obesity is preventable.

Obesity is a temporary state of being, if and only if you choose to eliminate it.

You have full control of what fuel you put in the tank, how much fuel, what properties of fuel, and what time of day for the fuel.

We can use these variables to our advantage and for one, *stop* gaining body fat, and two, *start* burning it off our bodies for fuel.

So again, what do you do now?

Well, that is why you're reading this book. Herein lies the secrets to successful weight loss, weight maintenance, and your life transformation. EXERLEAN will help you maximize your health and wellness and achieve your best quality of life forever!

I'm trying to wake you up! I'm trying to provoke a feeling in you, a drive to push you to make positive changes based on knowledge of the hardcore truth on the obesity predicament. I'm giving you ammunition to fight obesity, the power of awareness, and the beginnings of self-control. We are planting the seeds for success.

Remember, the goal with your fuel intake and with EXERLEAN in general is long-term lifestyle changes for the better. To always make the heavy-handed beneficial choices in life.

CHAPTER 8
Bodinomics: Work

OBESITY IS THE result of a twofold scenario. The main cause of obesity is overconsumption of food, but there is a lesser-contributing yet highly important factor: lack of physical activity or work.

I say "lesser-contributing" because it is well established in the bodybuilding, medical, and scientific community that what a person eats determines whether they will gain or lose body fat. This scenario of fuel versus activity is difficult to place a percentage on because every person is different, and the percentage fluctuates person to person. Based on my experience, I would state that 80 percent of gaining or losing body fat is the result of what we eat or don't eat, and 20 percent is the result of physical activity or work.

For example, a person can get totally ripped and ready for a bodybuilding show on 100 percent dieting alone. I've done it. However, there are negative consequences of dieting without exercise. As in loss of lean body mass, declining strength, less muscle tone, and deconditioning. I have also tried to get ripped for a show using exercise alone, and it 100 percent did *not* work. You can do ten hours of cardio and weight training a day, but if you're not eating restrictively, you will stay fat.

You will burn some body fat but then gain it back when you return to consuming or overconsuming unrestricted food choices.

So, why should you exercise if it plays a smaller role in body transformation than food restriction or dieting? Because the overall goal, after you earn your lean and toned body, is to achieve a state of maximal health and wellness for the long run. The division between the *EXER* and the *LEAN* in EXERLEAN is a fifty-fifty split. Exercise is vital in achieving a healthy state of physiology and homeostasis. Eating lean is necessary to stay lean. Exercise and work are necessary for organ health, maintaining general health and well-being, building and preserving lean body tissue, maximizing strength, conditioning, and maximizing fat burning. Exercise is a great tool to add to our arsenal in the transformation journey.

Being sedentary promotes obesity, weakness, diseases, and other negative health consequences. The human body needs to move. It thrives when it is active, moving, and exerting. Exerting is doing something that is physically stressful on the body, causing increased heart rate, respiratory rate, and calorie burning, or use of fuel. Being active and exerting helps our bodies use food for fuel, increases muscle tone, and improves circulation and cardiorespiratory conditioning.

Human beings have had to work for survival from the beginning of life. Hunting for food requires speed, agility, and endurance. Building shelter requires lifting, constructing, and moving heavy objects. Preparing food for preservation and meals takes manual labor. So does walking to get water from the source and carrying it home for use, and tilling and farming fields by hand for crops. Humans even had to make their own tools, clothing, and fixtures (and still do in some cultures). Up until the last century of human life, we have had it pretty tough. Nowadays with the benefits of science and technology, we barely have to move a muscle to accomplish the once-difficult goal of *survival*.

Because we no longer have to build our shelter or hunt, farm, and physically work for food, people are more sedentary than at any other time in human history. All we have to do is drive to the store and pay for food. And our jobs are increasingly less physically active and in fact very sedentary due to the rise in technology, automation, and machine-driven industries. Easy food and easy work. That is the predicament. We are eating and lounging ourselves to death.

The answer to the problem is supplementation. Not food supplementation. Supplementation of work. Since work is becoming less and less physically active, then we need to add in something else that is physical. We need to supplement work.

There are many options for lack of work. We just need to narrow it down to a few and focus on them with massive intensity and drive. Some employers offer employee fitness centers or will pay for an employee's gym membership. I would hope that someday most employers offer employee incentives to exercise at work, at a gym, at home, outside, or in a combination of all options. It is in the employer's best interest to help employees prevent and eliminate the obesity pandemic. Obesity leads to less productivity and therefore increased costs, which raises the employer's expense of the employee and leads to lower income or production for the business. Nobody wants to be the cog in the wheel or the chink in the chain.

Losing body fat is actually pretty easy.

Engaging in physical activity is too.

But believing it, and actually doing it, is a monumental hurdle for most people.

You can do anything if you believe in what you are doing. Envision future you, make a plan, set goals to achieve future you, and then attack the plan. Do the work with ferocity and tenacity!

Let's keep moving forward and figure out how to do this thing called transformation!

So, we have established that fuel and work are vital variables that we must manipulate, supplement, and control in order to achieve positive transformation. We can use the cost-benefit analysis to help us make decisions about food and activity. We know that we should always make the heavy-handed beneficial decision based on objective data derived from the CBA. This is how we can achieve our best potential within our own body's economy.

Let's dive a little more into the benefits of work, physical activity, sleep, eating, and play. How do we execute, manage, and perform our daily activities? Why does it matter how we perform these activities? Why are these activities so vital in determining our short- and long-term outcomes? Welcome to your healthstyle.

CHAPTER 9
Healthstyle

Life is the balancing act of survival, self-care, work, caregiving, love, play, sex, spirituality, eating, sleeping, and exercise.

We each have unique, precious, and important missions to accomplish during our time here on earth. To successfully complete a mission, we need to establish habits, then act out behaviors that will lead to successful outcomes. What aspects of life matter most on the journey to complete your healthstyle transformation?

We touched on healthstyle back in chapter 1. In contrast to your lifestyle, which involves everything about the way you live your life, your healthstyle is the daily routine, schedule, agenda, habits, and behaviors that dictate your present and future status—your success versus failure—in maintaining a healthy body weight, body fat composition, physical activity and exercise level, work productivity, play, eating, and sleeping.

We can modify our healthstyle and therefore burn more calories by changing the process of the simple daily activities we take for granted:

- What time do you wake up?
- Do you make your bed?
- Do you put your clothes out the night before?
- Do you prepare your meals for the week ahead of time?
- What do you do from the moment you wake until you go to sleep?
- When do you eat?
- When do you exercise?
- When do you work?

Does your schedule or routine promote obesity, disease, and progressive disability?

These and so many other factors play key roles in how successful you will be in reaching your goals. If your daily routine is full of wasted, sedentary, and unproductive time, then you will not reach your goals. If your daily routine is full of overconsumption, especially of calorie-dense processed foods, and devoid of nutritious vegetables and protein, then you will never accomplish your transformation goals. If you don't have scheduled times for exercise, leisure activity, and play, again, you will not achieve your transformation goals. The same outcome is true if you don't work. It is important for a person to feel needed and contribute to the fabric of society in some capacity. Work keeps people active and productive, which leads to increased calorie burning, increased activity, and expressing one's creativity.

Work takes on many different shapes and forms, from doctor to policeman, baker, homemaker, actor, NFL football player, volunteer, and author. The list of jobs humans can have is infinite.

Everyone has responsibilities, chores, and activities that need to be completed by the end of the day. We can break these into three major groups:

- Activities of daily living, or ADL
- Instrumental activities of daily living, or IADL
- Job status—employed, unemployed, self-employed, dependent, homemaker, parent, student, volunteer, retired, or disabled

How you schedule then execute the completion of ADL, IADL, and your job will determine the overall outcome, or reward versus regret, in your life. The quality in which you complete your ADL, IADL, and job are important attributes of your healthstyle.

So, what exactly are ADL, IADL, and jobs?

ADL (Activities of Daily Living)

ADL are composed of the simple basic tasks a person must complete for self-care. These self-care tasks include dressing, bathing, toileting, personal hygiene/grooming, self-feeding or eating, and functional mobility. These six tasks are crucial to remain self-sufficient and independent. If you are not self-caring, then why not? This is something you can change or work toward doing yourself.

Dressing includes putting on underwear, socks, pants, and shoes; tying shoes; looping a belt; donning a bra and shirt; threading your arms through the sleeves of a jacket or coat; and putting on a hat or hairpiece. Do you lay your clothing out at night, ready to don first thing in the morning? Do you put on your clothes with haste or at a snail's pace? Do you get dressed? If not, why?

Bathing or showering includes the process of getting in and out of the tub or shower, washing all your body parts with soap and water, rinsing off all the soap scum, then drying off with a towel. Is the result of your bathing task of high quality or low quality? Do you take long or short showers and baths? Do you bathe daily? If not, why?

Toileting includes a person's ability to get to the toilet, doff and don clothing, voiding oneself of urine and feces, then finally wiping and/or cleaning up oneself after urinating or having a bowel movement (BM). Do you take a long time at the toilet? Do you have difficulty cleaning yourself? How many BMs do you have in a day? Could your food type, quantity, and timing be playing a role in how many BMs you take in a day and whether they are loose, hard, or soft?

Remember, what goes in must come out, and if you are consuming garbage, then your body will reject most of it as waste and store the calories as body fat. If you are crapping all day long, then you are likely eating too much food of poor nutritional value. If you are eating lean, nutritious food in moderation, your body will use most of the calories for needed healing and other processes, resulting in less fat storage and less waste . . . or less poop!

Personal hygiene includes the lighter tasks of brushing your teeth and other oral care, grooming your hair, and hand and face washing. Do you brush your teeth? Do you groom your hair? Do you wash your hands after going to the bathroom, playing with pets, or working in dirt?

Self-feeding or eating is the simple task of moving food from dish to your mouth, chewing it up, and putting it in your belly. Do you eat slow, fast, too much, or too little? Do you spend too much time putting food in your mouth?

We only need enough food to repair and replace damaged cells, synthesize new lean body tissue, and provide fuel for our muscles, brain, and other organs. Any leftovers are going to body fat storage and waste.

Functional mobility includes the simple movements in life we take for granted until we can't do them anymore, like getting in and out of bed, standing up from the edge of bed or a chair, sitting down and getting off a toilet, stepping into and out of a shower or tub, walking from one end of the house to the other, going up and down stairs, and getting in and out of a car. Are you able to complete functional mobility? Do you move fast or slow? Is functional mobility easy or difficult for you?

IADL (Instrumental Activities of Daily Living)

Instrumental activities are not necessary for functional living but are associated with independent living and therefore improve your quality of life. IADL include house cleaning, laundry, cooking and meal prep, taking prescribed medications, money management and bill paying, communication via phone and internet, grocery shopping, driving, and community mobility, or the ability to walk around at a community level.

House cleaning is a lot of work. Vacuuming, mopping, scrubbing down sinks, toilets, and showers, doing the dishes, dusting, picking up, putting away clean clothes, organizing, and doing general upkeep take effort. Do you mope around or procrastinate when it comes to these cleaning tasks? If so, why?

Laundry is necessary to ensure having clean clothing to wear. Doing laundry can be a good form of exercise depending on how you complete the task.

Cooking and meal prep is obviously necessary for survival. If you eat out, get takeout, or order in for most of your meals, why? Did you know you can save money, eat healthier, and get more exercise by preparing your own meals?

Taking prescribed medications is necessary for some people to thrive or even survive. Do you take your prescriptions as your doctor has instructed? If not, why not? Did you know it is possible for some people to get off certain medications by adopting healthy eating habits, exercising regularly, and achieving a lean physique? Some people are on medications purely due to their sedentary behavior, poor eating habits, and morbid obesity. If you are one of these people, how about taking control of yourself and your actions with the goal of decreasing the burden of prescribed medications? Of course, this should be done under the guidance of your primary care doctor (MD) and with the coaching of a personal trainer and nutritionist.

Money management and bill paying is necessary to maintain residence in your home, keep the utilities on, and purchase groceries, gas, medications, and other necessities. If a person cannot manage money and budget for those necessities, then they will be unable to maintain independent living.

Communication nowadays is highly advanced. With texts, calls, and emails, we can communicate with one another on a level of ease and speed never before experienced in human history. We can now order our groceries, home essentials, and tools and even work from a smartphone. We can even talk to our smartphones. As the world of technology around us advances, so must we in order to thrive in our community, the economy, and society as a whole. Do you have a landline phone, a cell phone, a computer, or the internet? If not, why? How do you keep up with the world events, maintain socialization, and communicate with people who matter to you? What can you do to improve your social health?

Grocery shopping is vital for making meals at home, packing kids' lunches, preparing work lunches, and stocking up for busy times. If you don't go shopping for food, then you must be eating out. This is an expensive luxury, and unless you're eating low-calorie lean meals, it will lead to being overweight or obese over time. Do you eat out a lot? If so, why? Do you know how to go shopping? Do you know how to cook? If not, maybe it's time to start preparing meals at home. If you don't know how, learn!

Driving helps you take the kids to school, get to work, go to the grocery store, get to the gym, and easily socialize and move about in the community. Do you own a bike? Could you ride your bike to work for exercise? If you live close enough to work, you could walk. What can you do to decrease your dependency on driving and burn more calories? What about walking, riding a bike, Rollerblading, or skateboarding to your destination?

Community mobility is the chore of walking greater distances to accomplish tasks within your community. It includes tasks like making your way around a grocery store from the car, or walking around a shopping mall or through a movie theater or hospital. It is getting out and about for leisure, medical reasons, shopping, and really anything else outside your home. How can you improve your community mobility? Do you mobilize in your community? If not, why? What is stopping you? If you do, want to crank it up a notch? Go downhill skiing, trail hiking, or exploring.

Job Status

Aside from ADL and IADL, most of us work at a job for money in order to provide for ourselves and our family, or to contribute in some form to maintaining the status quo of the household or community. A person's job can vary from extreme manual labor to dead sedentary. Some jobs are high stress, some are low stress. Jobs can be fun and rewarding or boring and monotonous. Some are paying and some are nonpaying, but all jobs are necessary to live, survive, maintain the home, and contribute to the fabric of society.

When a person retires, becomes unemployed, or is disabled from work, there becomes a void. This void leads to sedentary behavior. It is vital to fill the void with some sort of activity to remain vibrant and moving to prevent the onset or progression of obesity, muscle atrophy, diseases, and disability. A person may need to get creative in figuring out how to fill that void depending on their unique situation.

Do you work? Do you have a purpose? Do you contribute to your household or to the community? If not, why, and what can you do to change the situation?

How you execute your ADL, IADL, and work contributes to your healthstyle. By moving faster and upping the intensity of your ADL, IADL, and job performance, you will burn more calories incrementally throughout your day. This in turn improves your healthstyle. For example, first thing in the morning, make your bed, and do it quickly. Take your shower faster. Put your clothes out the night before and get dressed faster than usual, which will also save you time. Some things, however, need to remain thorough, such as toileting, hair grooming, oral care, and hand and face washing. Look at all your self-care and morning-prep activities to see where you can shorten tasks and free up sedentary, valuable time for more productive endeavors that move you toward your life goals.

One example is spending less time applying makeup. You'll find you have more time for exercise, lean meal prep, and leisure activity.

The same applies to modifying your IADL to make these activities exercise. Do your laundry daily and move fast while you are doing it. Clean your home as fast as you can. Do your dishes by hand rather than the dishwasher. When you go shopping, don't use a power scooter, walk. If you normally walk, then walk faster to increase your calorie expenditure. Burn even more calories by parking at the far end of the parking lot to increase your walking distance. Same goes for any community mobility. Park further away and walk more.

Our work can also be modified to burn more calories by increasing movement, moving faster, or adding resistance. Park farther away, or consider riding a bike, walking, or jogging to work. If you have stairs at work, take the stairs rather than the elevator. Then advance toward taking double steps, going up the stairs faster, and taking the stairs during breaks. Speed-walk at work to burn more calories. If you have a desk job, see if your employer will get you a standing frame desk or treadmill desk, or if they'll allow walking or stair-climbing breaks as much as possible. If not, you can do chair squats every fifteen minutes. Add resistance by wearing ankle weights or a weight vest. Whatever your job, there are ways you can burn more calories. You just may need to get creative!

Modifying the way you complete simple self-care tasks, chores, or work tasks may seem silly or pointless, but consider this. All these ADL, IADL, and work activities are going to exist regardless of whether you modify your healthstyle. How you accomplish these daily tasks will determine whether you will harness the extra calorie-burning potential, which over time will make a positive difference overall.

For example, let's say you burn 80 calories in thirty minutes of average house cleaning. If you do it faster and with more intensity, then in the same thirty minutes, you can nearly double the number of calories you burn. You can easily burn 200–300 more calories a day by making similar healthstyle changes to your ADL, IADL, and work behavior. This free calorie burning will help you on the road to treating and preventing being overweight or obese. Your improved and efficient healthstyle will also make you more productive at home and work, freeing up more time for other things you've had no time to do, like go to the gym or engage in high-calorie-burning and strengthening exercise programs.

There are a few other important aspects of your healthstyle that we have not talked about yet. Caregiving, play, sex, spirituality, sleeping, eating, and exercise are vital to attaining heightened personal awareness. We are going to go into eating and exercise in depth in later chapters, but these other aspects of your healthstyle are also key factors that contribute to your weight, health, and wellness. So please, stay with me—do not be impatient and take the path of least resistance. These necessary skills will help you take care of yourself now and for the rest of your life.

Caregiving

Some of us are parents caring for children, and some of us are caring for our parents, other adults, or someone disabled or in a dependent status. Caregiving is a taxing, time-consuming, and rewarding occupation. Many caregivers do not self-care and neglect their personal needs, then reach a state of burnout, stress, and chronic fatigue. Whether you are a parent or other caregiver, it is vital that you make time to keep yourself happy and healthy. If you do not take care of yourself, your ability and quality of caregiving will suffer. As parents, we must lead by example.

Our kids will mimic and adopt our healthstyle. Do you want your kids to be sedentary, overweight, and unproductive? Then be that way yourself. If you are a poor example of health, then your kids are automatically starting out on the wrong foot, and unless they find other positive health role models at school or in other extracurricular activities, their chances of being obese in childhood or later in life are much higher.

Caregiving for a parent can be minimally to extremely difficult depending on their level of frailty, fall risk, and cognitive impairment, including dementia. If you are not maintaining your own health, happiness, and productivity, you should reconsider taking on the caregiver role to your parent, as you will burn out, stress out, and worsen your overall health, likely leading to failure. The good news is you can make positive healthstyle changes and prepare your body, mind, and spirit for the caregiver burden at hand.

Play

Smiling and laughing are positive and powerful personal attributes that can help us stay healthy and relieve stress. As we age, we smile less and less. According to Forbes, 30 percent of us smile more than twenty times a day, and less than 14 percent of us smile fewer than five times a day. Did you know that the average child smiles about four hundred times a day and laughs out loud about three hundred times a day? An adult laughs about seventeen times a day, much less than when play was the dominant occupation. According to the Mayo Clinic, "A good laugh has great short-term effects." Some of the effects are lightening your mental load and inducing actual physical responses in your body. Laughter can stimulate many organ functions, activate and relieve stress responses, and soothe tension. The long-term effects of laughter are improved immunity, decreased pain, enjoyment, and improved wellness.

Adults need to continue to play in order to maintain overall health and wellness. We should seek out things that will evoke smiles and laughter. Play is engaging in fun-loving, enjoyable, and personally rewarding activity. For me, it is being in God's country—going on a motorcycle ride, fishing, or camping in a national forest.

Taking in fresh air and enjoying the sound of nature, free from the stress of work and home life . . . ahh! What is your play activity? How can you change or arrange your schedule to spend more time in your play occupations?

Sex

Obviously it's exercise. Let's stop there.

Wellness and Spirituality

In all that you do on the path to achieving ultimate health and wellness, it is important to cater to the wellness of your entire being. Your wellness involves your thoughts, emotions, sense of well-being, or being centered—that is, emotionally stable and calm—in the universe. The journey of life can be a trial full of stressful, painful, and sad encounters. There will also be many happy, gratifying, rewarding, and peaceful moments. The ability to experience the good and tolerate the bad depends on your relaxation, recentering, and rethinking skills. There are many tools we can use to achieve this sense of balance.

Meditation is a popular activity to recenter oneself. Meditation is a repeated process of training your mind to focus and direct your thoughts toward centeredness and balance. Some of the benefits of meditation are to increase awareness of yourself and your surroundings, reduce anxiety, increase emotional health, improve quality of sleep, better your behavior and character, and help self-control or conquer addictions. Meditation can also provide other physical benefits like reduced pain or improved pain control and decreased blood pressure. Find peace!

In my view, prayer is likely the most common wellness activity practiced by most cultures of the world. Praying and praying often can provide peace of mind and forgiveness. Prayer can also help achieve physical, emotional, mental, and spiritual healing. Prayer can help a person feel a sense of belonging, a sense of higher power, and a sense of purpose. Prayer helps people make the right decisions and turn away from wrongdoing or evil. Prayer reminds us how to behave and helps us know when to turn the other cheek, to forgive and forget as appropriate.

Prayer can help you achieve a sense of great appreciation and grace. It can also help you find your center and balance the body, mind, and soul.

I believe you can use the power of your mind to help you achieve your dream body and life transformation. Many successful people use visualization as a tool to learn new skills, adopt new behaviors and habits, and form the environment of their dreams by believing in themselves and not giving a hoot what anyone else thinks. If you have not read *The Secret* by Rhonda Byrne or watched the movie, I highly recommend you do to help you understand more about this concept.

Sleep

How much sleep do you get? Is it quality sleep? Are you getting fat while you sleep?

The benefits of sleep are all aimed at replenishing, repairing, and resetting the body for another day of life's taxing ADL, IADL, and work. Another day of surviving your healthstyle.

For the purpose of your EXERLEAN transformation, I want you to focus on creating sleep habits that will help you burn body fat and revitalize for the next day. It is important to make sure you sleep well. To do this, you need to avoid stimulants in the second half of your wake cycle. For me and many others, this means no coffee, caffeine, herbal, or other chemical stimulants after lunch, but you will have to test the waters with your body, your sleep, and your healthstyle. Modify your healthstyle however you see fit to promote peaceful, restful, and quality sleep.

We all know about the benefits of sleep and that we're supposed to "make sure to get enough sleep." How much sleep you need, however, depends on your unique situation. Regardless of the number of hours, don't sleep any more than you need to, and avoid sleep deprivation. Sleeping too much or too long will lead to negative health results, including increased risk of metabolic problems, adult onset diabetes, heart disease, lethargy, and obesity. A survey completed by the National Institutes of Health, "The Risks of Sleeping 'Too Much,'" concluded that in the general population, sleeping too much is associated with increased risk of psychiatric diseases and obesity/higher body mass index (BMI).

Sleeping too much can also lead to increased fatigue, chronic fatigue, lethargy, depression, and death.

Whoa! There it is again . . . death. It is astonishing that negative behavior and healthstyle choices can actually facilitate our early demise. Well, good thing you're becoming self-aware of this and taking action to end the onset-of-early-death dilemma! Who would have thought you can sleep yourself to death!

Taking control of your sleep pattern is a key aspect of the EXERLEAN program. The goal here is to adopt an adequate but not excessive quality sleep routine. Not only that, but by creating the right sleep environment through strategic presleep nutrition and timing, it is possible to create a state of fat burning during sleep. I call it *fasted sleep*. The first goal of fasted sleep is to prevent storing body fat during sleep. The second goal is to create a state of thermogenic sleep—that is, burning off body fat *while you are sleeping*.

One of the main contributors to obesity is consuming a meal directly before going to sleep. When you are sleeping, the last thing in the world your body needs is a gut full of calories, or energy. Any energy unconsumed for activity will be stored as body fat.

We can actually incinerate more body fat at night sleeping than when awake. Because the body does not have any calories in the stomach to use for energy, this leaves only body fat or lean muscle tissue to break down for energy. By not eating two or three hours before bed—essentially fasting—you can achieve weight loss. By this one action alone, you can begin a weight loss journey. We'll talk more about storing and expending energy later in the book.

Adopting a positive, calorie-burning, and productive healthstyle is an important first step in your EXERLEAN transformation. How you behave, move, and act out your ADL, IADL, and work is the foundation of your overall health and wellness now and for the rest of your life. So, start making changes to your ADL, IADL, and work processes, and you'll burn more calories and increase your productivity at home and at work—before even starting an exercise or dieting program.

PART 2

The "EXER" in EXERLEAN

EXERLEAN: Resolution for the physique transformation of a lifetime.

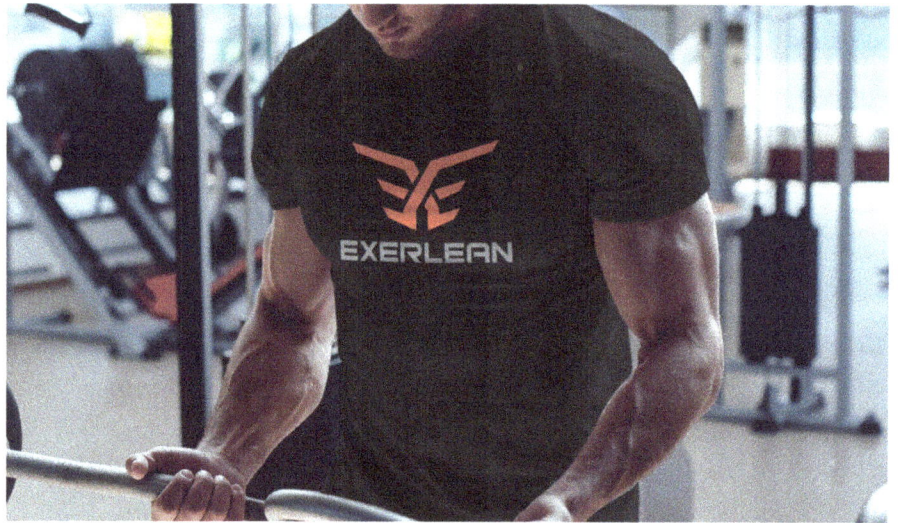

The EXERLEAN logo represents 6-Pack abs.
Two "E's" mirrored... "E"xerlean

Like the superman crest for hope
6-pack abs are a badge of honor

CHAPTER 10
EXERLEAN

We just learned about Bodinomics—the economy of the human body—and how to use the cost-benefit analysis to help us make the heavy-handed beneficial decisions dealing with food, activity, and any other decision that will move us forward in this transformation. We discussed our healthstyle and how we can modify our behavior and performance in all aspects of life, from dressing, bathing, and toileting to home chores, meal prep, and shopping to our jobs, roles, and contribution to society. By modifying our healthstyle, we can create a fat-burning exercise environment as we engage in ADL, IADL, and work just by moving faster, upping the intensity, and using the power of the mind—envisioning future you.

Finally, we tuned in to an important tool or state of fat burning called fasted sleep. By eating and timing our nutrition correctly, we can prevent storing body fat and create a thermogenic environment while we lie sedentary at night . . . burning off body fat in our sleep!

The key feature of Bodinomics, healthstyle, and fasted sleep is that they are all free. No gym membership required. No special foods. No supplements. No need to find time to do them. They are all part of what you are already doing; we are just changing the way we do them and the way we think about them.

We are preparing the body for mental, physical, and spiritual change. Preparing it for what you believe you can achieve. It is time to establish a new perspective, a vision of future you, and focus on the prize. I want you to do everything with an in-it-to-win-it attitude. I want you to "run in such a way that you may win" (1 Corinthians 9:24–26). This in-it-to-win-it attitude and running-in-such-a-way-that-you-may-win mindset should subsume you throughout your day and in every activity you engage in.

From here on, we are going to establish the essential knowledge and skills you need to take control of your body, habits, and behaviors to successfully transform your body, mind, and spirit. You are now going to learn everything necessary to change yourself into a healthy, lean, strong, and sexy sculpted you. Pay attention, memorize, learn, and absorb the materials, tools, and processes you will need to put into practice to win the war on body fat, weakness, and deconditioning.

EXERLEAN is a way of living. It is the incorporation of exercising, living lean, and contributing in every aspect to our existence. According to Newton's third law of motion, for every action, there is an equal and opposite reaction. The outcome—your results—will equal the input, or work, that you deliver to the entire transformative process.

The chapters ahead will give you the necessary tools to win your new body and new way of life.

I have included the somewhat complex, most efficient secrets to success that competitive bodybuilders, fitness competitors, actors, and models use to chisel their bodies into perfection and win the game of body transformation.

Competitive bodybuilders are able to achieve fat burning, or thermogenesis, at an unbelievable level compared to the average dieter. Why is this? It is because the competitor has learned the necessary knowledge dealing with the science of nutrition and how their bodies react to and change in certain nutritional environments. They have adopted a motive to get bigger muscles for bodybuilding and competing on stage. To get bigger muscles, they weight train to tear down muscle tissue, provoking the body to rebuild bigger and stronger, which in turn increases their metabolism and makes fat burning even easier.

EXERLEAN takes the secrets bodybuilders use to get lean fast and incorporates them into your program. It also incorporates the premise of bodybuilding—that by building more lean body mass, you also increase your metabolism, thus making fat burning easier during life. Therefore, weight training is a key tool for improving your muscle strength and size and ultimately, your fat-burning metabolism.

Now, I'm not talking about getting superhuman huge. That is

impossible. Worrying about getting too big or looking too muscle-bound is a waste of your time. Bodybuilders train for years and years at an intensity level unimaginable to the average person to gain a noticeable amount of new muscles. If you gain any amount of lean body mass during your EXERLEAN transformation, then consider it a blessing or a win because you are stronger and have an improved fat-burning machine under your skin.

You are going to learn about the benefits of exercise and how weight training, cardio, and living an active lifestyle are necessary to gain and maintain health, wealth, and longevity. Wait—wealth? Yeah, I call it "health and wealthness": the combination of health, wealth, and wellness all in one. We will talk about how health and wellness leads to improved wealth-generating potential and vice versa—how being wealthy helps you be healthy and well. They feed on each other, complement each other. True happiness in life cannot be fulfilled without maximizing one's health, wellness, and spirituality and having enough wealth to support your desired lifestyle.

We are about to delve into the benefits of weight training, how to do it, and when. Weight training is necessary for maintaining bone density and growth, joint support and stability, motor recruitment, and damage then repair of muscle tissue. Weight training improves one's overall muscle tone, strength, and power. The benefits of weight training also lead to improved self-confidence, mood, focus, and energy.

EXERLEAN *Chaining* or *Weight Chaining*, derived from my experience in the world of acute care occupational therapy, is a weight training program I have designed based on the anterior chain muscle groups (all the muscles in the front of your body) and posterior chain muscle groups (all the muscles in the back of your body).

The process of chaining promotes extension and helps fight the long-term effects of gravity in slowly pulling us closer to the earth over the course of our lives. Weight Chaining comes in three phases: beginner/low threshold, intermediate/moderate threshold, and extreme athlete/competitive bodybuilder, powerlifter, and professional athlete.

The benefit of Chaining is that you can hit all your muscles in as few as two efficient workouts a week. The chaining process can save you time and productivity in the long run depending on your personal goals and ambitions.

Fasted cardio is likely the most beneficial fat-burning tool at your disposal. You will learn what it is, how to do it, and the benefits of fasted cardio in the coming chapters.

EXERLEAN will help you acquire a physiological state of body fat incineration referred to as *the State* using the processes of Chaining, fasted cardio, and many other well-known exercise techniques to successfully complete your physical transformation. Don't forget about adapting your healthstyle, harnessing the benefits of fasted sleep, and using the Bodinomics: cost-benefit analysis in decision-making.

The first few chapters on the obesity epidemic, the Obesiboomers, and the preposterous disaster of poor or no butt wiping gave you the stun gun, cattle prod, slap in the face, or wakeup call necessary to self-actualize your situation and start planning for change. It's time to move on to the *EXER* in EXERLEAN and then the *LEAN*, helping you win your new body and complete your healthstyle transformation.

"Let's do this!"

CHAPTER 11
The Benefits of Exercise

THE NUMBER ONE path to fat burning is through calorie restriction and strategic dieting. But when it comes to achieving overall health and wellness for a lifetime, exercise is the number one tool at your disposal. Say hello to the *EXER* in EXERLEAN. It's half the formula for living in a healthy body for life. When we hear the word "exercise," we automatically think of it as working out on some sort of designated exercise equipment like a treadmill, elliptical trainer, or recumbent bike. These are all great forms of exercise but only a drop in the water glass. There are many forms of exercise in variable intensities, workloads, and leisure value; these depend on how much energy you exert in a certain amount of time. Daily healthstyle activities like doing laundry, cleaning the house, and doing yardwork are forms of exercise depending on the speed in which you move. Hiking on a trail, rowing a boat on a pond, paddling a canoe in the river are forms of exercise depending on the difficulty, environment, and other variables. Running and jogging are exercise due to the obvious increase in workload beyond our comfort zone, but they will have different outcomes depending on the setting, physical output, environmental resistance, and other variables.

Walking can be exercise if it's long enough and if you add in higher-workload variables, like walking uphill and downhill, wearing a weighted backpack, or walking fast. Really anything other than being sedentary can be considered exercise depending on the person's conditioning, especially in morbidly obese deconditioned individuals.

Sedentary behavior is the enemy of all of us. It leads to weight gain, deconditioning, weakness, and poor health. We must replace sedentary behavior with active behavior that works toward the ultimate goal: to have the least amount of sedentary behavior from the moment we wake up to the time we go to bed, for the rest of our lives.

So, how can we change sedentary behavior into exercise behavior?

First, let's change your deathstyle into a healthstyle.

The process starts from the moment you wake up. Take control of your body, environment, and self-care from the get-go. First, make your bed. Don't procrastinate. Just get it done rapidly and with tenacity. Keep up with this rapid process, task to task, while getting ready for the day. Don't sit down first thing. You just finished sleeping all night long! The last thing you need is to rest after being dead sedentary the last seven to eight hours. Hell, no—you need to earn your rest. Rest is the reward or necessary tool for recovery after work. So, until you work enough to earn rest, keep moving and don't stop.

Execute your ADL, IADL, and job as though you are walking on fire. If you have free time, add in another activity, and another, and so on. Just because you freed up some extra time by moving faster and getting things done early does not warrant sedentary behavior.

What kind of activities can you do with your newly etched-out free time? Watch TV?

Wrong!

Come on, now; get excited and creative with your free time! The list of possibilities is infinite.

The difference between the richest and most successful people, including star athletes, and the rest of us is they do not waste time with nonproductive activities unless they have planned them for leisure and reward. They work in a way that most of us cannot fathom. They move and work constantly, complete projects repeatedly, and when free time arises, they fill it with the next planned project or work. This behavior paves the way to wealth in many areas of life.

We can mimic the behavior of the rich and successful to achieve better outcomes in our own lives. We can incorporate those behaviors to develop our bodies and otherwise build out our individual empires. If you get all your self-care, chores, and work done and have some free time left, you can fill it with something productive toward your transformation goals, like exercising. Get on a treadmill, go to the gym, get outside and go hiking, ride a bike, or hit the punching bag. Get wild and creative with your free time. For now, you need to dedicate this extra time to fat loss, but down the road when you have achieved your dream body and healthstyle transformation, you can explore other exciting productive activities. Write a book, start a side business, build a website, knit a blanket, paint the house, or complete any other endeavor of passion. Until then, it is vital to fill your free time with exercise or other active leisure activities to maintain the momentum of your transformation.

Your life depends on it.

First your health, then the pursuit of happiness.

The time frame for a healthstyle and body transformation is individualized. It will depend on your unique life circumstances and goals. Regardless, from the beginning you need to visualize your end goal. What does future you look, feel, and function like?

When you attain that future vision, when it manifests in the flesh, you have reached the ultimate goal. To keep it, you will need to move to a maintenance phase. Maintenance of your final product. Future you has now become present you, and keeping it is vital.

Every person has a unique life with individualized and shared responsibilities. Depending on whether you are a stay-at-home parent, go to work, go to school, work at home, or fit into another scenario, you have opportunities to exercise throughout the day. You will have to get creative, move faster, and adopt an active healthstyle. As we've mentioned, if you have a sedentary job, add in exercise whenever you can. Keep a couple of dumbbells under your desk to do a five-to-ten-minute workout every couple of hours, go up and down a flight of stairs throughout the day, and speed-walk on your lunch break. It is up to you to create active opportunities. Ask your employer for help. Employers know that healthy employees are happy employees and are more productive in the long run.

Exercise does so many different things to the human body. By taking the body out of its resting state, it forces the body to start working—the heart rate goes up, blood circulates faster and is delivered to all areas of the body, the brain increases alertness, and every cell prepares for metabolism. Let's look at the body's response to exercise in more detail.

Cardiac—Circulation, Blood Pressure, and Heart Rate

When muscles are in a resting state, 20 to 25 percent of the capillaries are open and moving blood. When exercising, 100 percent of your body's capillaries are open and transporting blood, delivering vital nutrients to all areas of the body. Exercise increases heart rate and stroke volume (the amount of blood that passes through the heart in one beat), thus elevating overall cardiac output. Cardiac output is the combination of heart rate, blood pressure, and stroke volume. Heart rate is the number of times your heart beats in a minute. Blood pressure is when the blood supply flows from high-pressure areas to low-pressure areas—meaning from the heart outward to the farthest areas of the body. The quality of nutrient delivery depends on several factors, including cardiac output, blood volume, and the circulatory system. If a person has peripheral vascular disease (PVD), peripheral artery disease (PAD), or some other impairment of their veins and arteries comprising the circulatory system, then delivering nutrients to the farthest reaches of the body will be impaired.

The good news is exercise can help a person prevent further pruning of their veins and arteries and possibly improve their circulatory system by creating more supply branches of capillaries and venules (smaller blood vessels) to deliver nutrients to the farthest reaches of the body. Research has proven over and over again that exercise results in an overall benefit on improving cardiac output and circulation, as well as preventing heart and peripheral vascular disease.

Respiration—Lung Function and Breathing

During exercise, we begin to breathe deeper and more often to deliver oxygen to body tissues, then we transport and exhale carbon dioxide. Our body's conditioning to exercise or work determines how our lungs function. The more active and athletic a person's healthstyle, the better conditioned and efficient their system is at delivering oxygen and picking up carbon dioxide throughout the body. A healthy or conditioned person will have a lower overall respiratory or breath rate per minute than a deconditioned person. That is why a deconditioned person will huff and puff during exercise, whereas a conditioned or healthy person will have an unnoticeable change in respiratory rate doing the exact same exercise at the same rate.

As you change your body during your transformation, at some point you will notice that you can endure longer and higher-difficulty exercise sessions without huffing and puffing as your conditioning improves.

Metabolism

Metabolism is the rate at which the body assimilates food, turns food into energy, and expends energy. All foods are made up of chemical substances. How a person's body handles the total of all chemical changes results in either an anabolic or catabolic metabolism pathway.

Anabolism is a process that uses energy to join smaller molecules into larger ones. It helps all tissues, hormones, and neurotransmitters in our bodies to grow, synthesize, replenish, and repair. Anabolism helps build our body, which is why it requires energy or fuel. For the purpose of your EXERLEAN transformation, anabolic metabolism should simply be thought of as growth and repair in our bodies.

There are four major hormones that have anabolic properties: insulin, testosterone, human growth hormone, and estrogen. All cause the body to grow, gain, store, or develop. We will focus on insulin in particular in this book.

In anabolism, there is a very bad possible outcome—storage of body fat. As a state of growth, anabolism is good when it comes to repairing and growing lean body mass or muscle tissue, but it's bad if an excess of calories is not burned off during work; it will store those calories as body fat.

#fatback is what occurs when you burn off body fat and then gain it back again. This is the worst scenario of going on a weight loss plan. #fatback is usually the result of cheating or deviating from the program. If you're not cheating, you have accidentally miscalculated and therefore overconsumed calories. Your body has mixed signals during restrictive dieting and thinks it's starving, so it will store any excess calories for survival. If you don't have excess calories, you don't have any that can get stored as body fat. That's why it is vital that you do not cheat during a fasting state—it will reverse progress by causing you to regain body fat you worked so hard to lose. This leads to lower self-esteem, lower self-confidence, and a higher likelihood of quitting altogether. *Never* throw in the towel. We learn from mistakes and come back stronger as a result.

Catabolism is the process of breaking down larger molecules into smaller molecules, releasing energy as a result. Catabolism starts with digestion and ends in cellular tissues of the body. The energy derived from catabolism is used to facilitate anabolic reactions. For the purpose of your EXERLEAN transformation, catabolic metabolism should simply be thought of as the breakdown or destruction of our body tissues and a process that releases energy or fuel for the body to use. The breakdown of skeletal muscle (#eatmuscles) and the destruction of body fat are catabolic. A way I like to think of catabolism in the human body is with a similar word, cannibalism. A catabolic pathway in our body is in a way eating ourselves alive. For the purpose of your EXERLEAN transformation, you should strive to put your body into a state of metabolizing your body fat, glycogen, and food for fuel and *not* your muscles.

#eatmuscles is what occurs if not you're consuming enough protein or calories to maintain lean body mass when you're in a state of continuous fasting and exercise and/or restrictive dieting and fat burning.

We want to harness the thermogenic properties of body fat incineration and at all costs avoid the breakdown of our valuable skeletal muscle tissue.

Remember: your resting metabolic rate (RMR)—the rate at which you burn calories when your body is at rest—is based on the amount of skeletal muscle you have; therefore, it is vital to maintain and increase muscle mass as much as possible. Increasing muscle mass results in positive outcomes, namely improved strength, increased power, and higher resting metabolic rate, that will help you succeed in your transformation.

Endorphins

Exercise triggers the release of *endorphins*, or the good-vibes hormones, which results in an elated mental state, an acute increase in cognitive awareness, and an overall positive sense of well-being. Endorphins, neurochemicals produced in the pituitary gland, are predominantly released into the bloodstream to treat pain and stress by reacting with the opiate receptors in your brain, just like narcotic painkillers, alcohol, cocaine, and amphetamines do. Naturally occurring endorphins are healthy; those from synthetic substances are not.

Prescription painkiller overdosing linked to unintentional death is now the number one preventable cause of death in the United States. Alcohol is an over-the-counter beverage with obvious benefits and negative outcomes depending on the amount consumed and whether it is abused or an addiction. Cocaine and amphetamines are illegal and highly addictive drugs that destroy people's lives. All these drugs release endorphins into the bloodstream and create positive mood-altering effects and therefore habit and addiction. Since exercise also releases endorphins, it should lead us to think that exercise should be the number one weapon in the treatment plan to overcome these addictions. For the purposes of your EXERLEAN transformation, we will stick with getting our endorphins from exercise!

Exercise promotes a ready state in all the cells of your body. It positively affects your heart, lungs, brain, other organs, and mind. This ready state helps manage stress, pain, and depression. When all your cells are activated, it also jacks your metabolic state and helps burn off calories and body fat for the remainder of the day. Exercise and weight training also help with hormone modulation and can impact your mental health by improving self-confidence, mood, and your general mental state.

The endorphin release during exercise is long lasting and will help maintain a positive mood so you feel energized and ready to tackle the world. Because of this, it is beneficial to get your cardiovascular exercise first thing in the morning. Talk about getting your foot out the door on a positive note.

Exercise is natural and within our control. Exercising daily can help people prevent and manage type 2 diabetes, reduce risks of some cancers, improve overall longevity, maintain and improve sexual function, improve sleep quality, help smokers quit smoking, strengthen bones, strengthen muscles, improved balance, and decrease risk of falling. Exercise is one of the healthiest, if not the healthiest, treatments for obesity, diseases, and many disabilities, so it should always be considered the first medicine.

CHAPTER 12
Weight Training

We know now the benefits of exercise for improved physical health, weight loss, and an overall sense of well-being. Well, what weight training can do for the human body is comparable to the fountain of youth. Weight training is your activity of choice to promote longevity and stem the effects of aging. Weight training results in increased muscle tone, higher power, increased metabolic rate, stronger bones, improved athletic performance, better mobility, improved diabetes outcomes, treatment and prevention of musculoskeletal pain and deformity, improved balance, and improved mental health. Weight training also helps fight off osteoporosis, muscle atrophy, cardiovascular deconditioning, falls, bone demineralization, obesity, the effects of aging, cognitive impairment, and dementia.

I want to keep weight training as simple as possible to help you win the war against body fat so you can attain the greatest physique of your life. In the world of dieting, exercise, and weight training, the jargon can get very confusing if you are not an athletic trainer or a healthcare professional, or if you aren't well read on anatomy and physiology of the human body. That's why I will follow up complicated words with easy descriptors—for example, "anterior quadriceps," or front upper-leg muscles.

EXERLEAN follows the rule of KISS—keep it simple, silly!

So, What Exactly Is Weight Training?

What makes weight training different from exercise? Well, weight training is exercise, just a resisted and anaerobic form of it. Exercise we typically think of like jogging, swimming, running, and using an elliptical, stair-stepper, or exercise bike are all aerobic exercise. *Aerobic* means "with oxygen," as in when you exercise aerobically, you need to breathe and supply direct oxygen for the exercise. *Anaerobic*—meaning without oxygen—exercise requires lower cardiorespiratory effort and therefore does not require extra oxygen other than what is normally necessary to breathe for life.

To give you a good example, imagine running as fast as you can for thirty seconds. If you're like most people, at the end you will bend over with your hands on your knees taking in deep and rapid breaths, or you'll at least be huffing and puffing. Weight training rarely leads to this shortness-of-breath result, unless it is done with very high reps. Aerobic exercise is typically done without any resistance or extra weight and also at a longer duration or bout of exertion, whereas anaerobic exercise uses weight resistance and is completed in sets of lower repetitions. For EXERLEAN, we will always consider weight training an anaerobic exercise unless otherwise specified.

Simply put, weight training involves picking stuff up, moving it around, and putting it back down. The heavier the stuff, the better! It involves a certain number of sets per weight-resisted exercise and a certain number of repetitions per set.

The Secrets of Successful Weight Training

When most people think of weight training, they picture bodybuilders, powerlifters, or Hollywood actors like Kate Beckinsale, Dwayne "The Rock" Johnson, Halie Berry, or Chris Hemsworth. Well, they look sexy and strong, right? Why not follow suit?

Bodybuilders discovered the secrets and benefits of weight training far before the medical industry did. We've said it before—when it comes to burning off body fat and getting ripped, a seasoned bodybuilder knows the secret sauce. The best, most useful information for weight training that actually works comes from a bodybuilding expert with knowledge, experience, and proof of concept in attaining a shredded body composition. Same can be said for gaining lean muscle mass or building muscle bulk. As an expert with twenty-two years of bodybuilding and dieting experience, I know weight training is a vital weapon in your arsenal in the fight against obesity, whether it's four hundred pounds or thirty pounds you need to lose.

Before we talk about how to weight train, let's discuss some preconceived misconceptions.

For one, it is seriously hard to gain muscle mass, so quit worrying about getting too big or looking too muscular. That mindset will hold you back.

Remember, lean body mass or muscle tissue determines your resting metabolic rate and ability to burn off body fat. The more muscle you have, the more you can eat and the easier it is to get lean. So if you gain some muscles during your transformation, then you should be jumping for joy if anything.

Two, it is difficult to gain muscle mass doing aerobic exercises, and since adding muscle mass is so beneficial in the fight against obesity, then weight training, which is anaerobic, is an important tool you must take advantage of. In fact, it should be your preferred exercise regimen.

Remember: dieting is the number one way to lose body fat, basically through starvation. It's starvation of energy derived from food, then forcing your body to burn body fat for energy to work. Weight training basically increases your fat-burning metabolism by growing more muscles. Weight training in the least helps maintain current muscle bulk and prevents muscle catabolism—the worst outcome possible when dieting since muscle loss equals lower metabolism.

Weight training can be completed in many ways. You might picture yourself or someone else working out in a gym environment, but weight training can take place basically anywhere. You can weight train in your yard, at home, at work, at the gym, or in a park. You may just need to be creative. For example, pull-ups and push-ups are resisted exercise and are therefore weight training using body weight. In the kitchen, you can use a couple of soup cans as weights for biceps curls, shoulder presses, triceps extensions, and squats. You get the idea!

One repetition max, or 1RM in weight lifting refers to the heaviest weight a person can lift through full range of motion during a particular exercise for one repetition. Power lifting competitions revolve around this concept. She or he who lifts the most weight wins. Most typical workouts work towards the heaviest possible 1RM on the last set of the exercise. Many designer workout programs start out with and advance based on a person's one rep max. To figure this out there are a few 1RM formulas that help you figure out where to start and end the resistance levels of your workout. This process is complicated; therefore it is helpful to have a coach or personal trainer help you figure this out. If you want to tackle this on your own, there is a one rep max calculator that you can use at www.bodybuilding.com.

The key to successful outcomes with weight training is to do as much resistance weight as possible—so the heavier, the better—and maintain good body mechanics. Then you need to use that weight and do enough sets and repetitions (reps) to break down or strain your muscles, which in turn demands a response from your body to reinforce itself to be better prepared for the next bout of work.

Muscle breakdown is achieved by resisting a heavy enough weight through sets of repetitions to achieve a state called *hypertrophy*, or *muscle pump*. We all have heard of "getting pumped up," right? Arnold Schwarzenegger is known for saying, "I'm going to pump you up!" He has also referred to the muscle pump as being better than an orgasm.

When a muscle has received enough workload through repetitions and sets using weight resistance, the muscles will eventually become swollen and bigger. This is the result of the body sending nutrient-rich blood to the muscles being stressed. The muscle pump is a sign that the area of the body being trained is now warmed up and poised for a maximum onslaught of heavy work.

When in a state of muscle hypertrophy, the effort or work being exerted actually feels good. You feel better, stronger, relieved. The leaner you are, the more you can feel a muscle pump, and the more you can see the difference. What I mean by this is that if you are covered in a thick layer of body fat, then you will feel the muscle pump, but it will not really be noticeable in the mirror. You may look a bit bigger overall, but you won't have the ripped look a bodybuilder attains from a combination of being lean (little to no body fat) and the temporary state of a muscle pump. Regardless of whether you are fat or lean, the muscle pump achieved from lifting weights is incredible. Although your swollen muscles will shrink down to normal size within hours, the increased muscle tone can last for days.

In the EXERLEAN program, the muscle pump is the goal of weight training, and when you achieve a muscle pump, you'll add weight and go to town on the sets and reps. This will lead to positive physical change through increased muscle tone, strength, and if lucky, more lean body mass during the recovery phase.

So, how do you do this thing called weight training? For beginners, working out in general may seem overwhelming and complicated. More often than not, a beginner or inexperienced weightlifter's fear will lead them to quit before they even give it a fair chance. For one, you have the difficulty of breaking a bad behavior, which is *not* working out. Add to that learning a new, unhabituated activity. Breaking bad habits and forming new ones takes effort, time, and discipline. Learning a new skill takes dedication, perseverance, and fortitude to make it stick.

You can break sedentary habits and adopt new active habits. You can learn the skill of exercise, weight training, and in general working out and make these behaviors habitual in your life.

Believe it or not, weight training or working out is not complicated. To be successful, all you have to do is move weight around in sets of repetitions. *It is that easy!* It seems more complicated at first because there are thousands of different variations, names, formats, protocols, and programs out there being advertised. Don't let all these different ways to work out scare you off. All these exercise programs, including those in the EXERLEAN program, do the same thing. Your body needs to move, exert, and work against a resisting force. You can use metal weight plates and barbells, dumbbells, kettlebells, machines, weight stacks, resistance bands, medicine balls, body weight, Bodyblades, weighted vests, wrist or ankle weights, and anything else that achieves the same goal: exerting against an outside force that makes your body work hard, reach muscle pump, cause tissue breakdown, and then recover stronger-better-faster with good nutrition and rest.

The Physiology of Weight Training

Now, before we get into the basics of weight training and how to do it, let's lay out what happens with the body during your workouts first.

The body has over six hundred named muscles. To get started with weight training, we only need to know six major muscles groups and body parts: arms, shoulders, chest, abdominals, back, and legs. Each body part has a location—right or left, distal (far away) and proximal (close to the body), anterior (front) and posterior (backside), top (cephalic) and bottom (caudal), inside (medial) and outside (lateral). A simple exercise movement usually involves many of these six muscle groups or parts working together. That's why weightlifters do not need to get into individual little areas of the body beyond these six unless they are competitive bodybuilders looking to balance out the symmetry or aesthetics of their physique, or for rehabilitation of an injury or muscle imbalance under the guidance of a physical or occupational therapist.

A whole-body workout can be completed with a leg exercise, a chest exercise, a shoulder exercise, an arm exercise, and back and abdominal exercises, each exercise incorporating both the left and right side of your body at the same time. You will just need to do enough sets and reps with enough weight to tax your body enough to force it to respond with a good muscle pump, muscle tissue breakdown, and strengthening. So if you're a minimalist and the *least-resistive path* is your healthstyle, then there you go. But if you're looking for the maximum reward or benefit of weight training and desire to get as much as you can out of your work, then we need to delve a little deeper down the rabbit hole.

Let's go through each of the six areas of the body.

Arms

Arms are often the body part people think to exercise first. The arm can be broken up into the hands, forearms, biceps, and triceps. The hand is operated by the muscles in the forearm for grabbing and letting go of things. Your hand moves toward your body when your bicep contracts, or flexes. Your hand is pushed away from your body when your tricep contracts. The arm has many motions; the shoulder, elbow, wrist, and digits extend and contract; and your hand grips and releases.

To get a great arm workout, you must complete a weight training exercise for the biceps and triceps—the bis and tris—which coincidentally will also work out the forearm. The forearm also gets worked out in back, chest, and shoulder workouts. So we don't need to do the forearms in an arm workout. Half the arm workout is biceps, and the triceps is the other.

Biceps: The biceps are often the first muscle a person will gravitate toward working out at the gym. I mean, when someone wants to show a sign of strength, what do they do? Flex their arm up in the air and

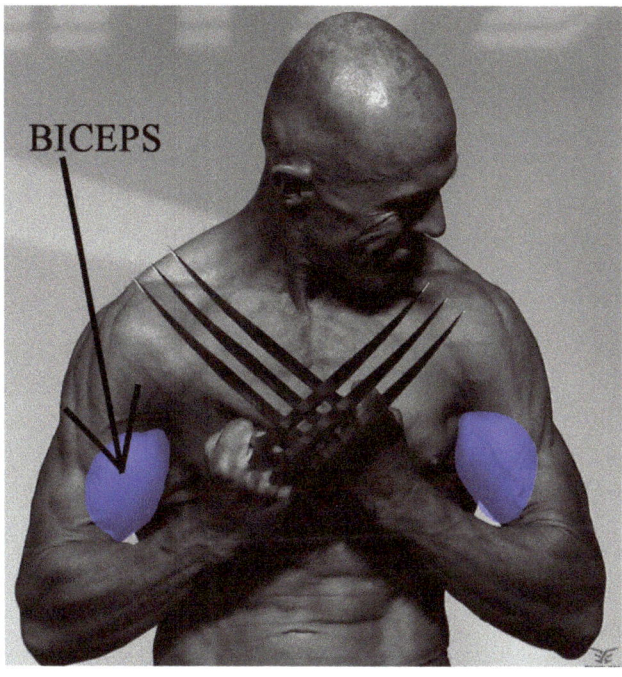

contract that bicep. The Popeyes, I like to call them. Some call them their guns. If you want to be great at tug-of-war, then work your biceps because they're responsible for pulling things toward your body. In a bodybuilding competition, the "front double biceps" pose, usually with a leg extended, is a mandatory pose.

The first and foremost weight training exercise for the bicep is the curl. To do a rep, grab on to a dumbbell, kettlebell, bar, or machine and move your hands from arms extended to arms closed, pulling the resistance closer to you. Hold it for a pause, then release to full extension, getting ready for the next rep. Then complete as many reps and sets as it takes to achieve a muscle pump and exhaust the muscle being worked. Typically, four to six sets of ten to fifteen reps with a couple-minute break between each set will achieve the muscle pump, or muscle hypertrophy.

Doing just one exercise per body part is enough, but it's not the best format. If you do just one weight training exercise per body part, then you have to do high sets and reps—or increased *volume*—of that exercise. Enough to reach muscle pump, muscle fiber damage, and muscle fatigue or exhaustion. Preferably, you should break all those sets into different exercises of smaller sets to stimulate the body part or area you're working with variability and differentiation, which prevents your body from adapting to the exercise and results in reaching "muscle annihilation" quicker. This goes for all body parts in your EXERLEAN weight training program.

Triceps

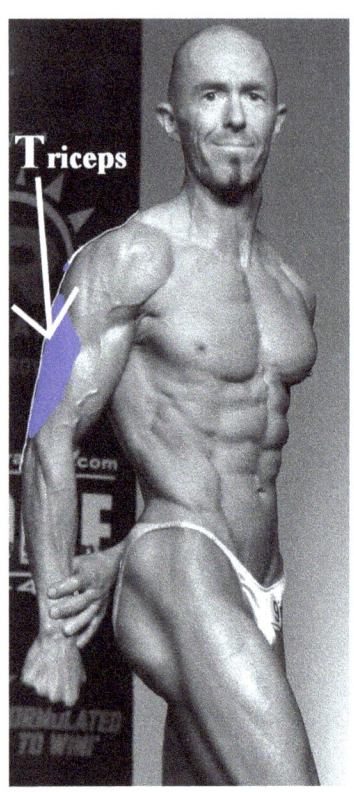

The triceps are greatly misrepresented. People assume that big muscular arms are due to biceps size when in reality, the triceps are responsible for two-thirds of the arm size. So if you want to increase the muscularity of your arms, then focusing on your triceps will get you there faster than working your biceps. Triceps size is a make-or-break detail in muscle aesthetics and bodybuilding competitions. Look at a picture of Arnold Schwarzenegger flexing his arms. The triceps are two-thirds of his arm, yet his biceps always get the credit. The "side triceps" pose, with same-side leg extended opposing knee flexed, then hands clasped behind the back, is a mandatory bodybuilding pose.

Because the triceps push things away from the body, if you want to be a great football lineman, you should maximize triceps strength and size to gain that extra edge in pushing your opponent away with the thrust of a jackhammer. A tennis player uses triceps during a serve and backswing to push the ball away from the body using a racket. The triceps are the key muscles used when a carpenter hammers a nail. They're very functional in many of life's activities.

The most common weight training exercises for triceps include close-grip bench press, cable push-downs, dumbbell kickbacks, dips, skull crushers, and overhead extensions.

Forearms

Although the forearm gets its main workout from heavier compound movements during the chest and back workouts, if you want to add a third exercise to focus on your forearms, then a grip spring or grip strengthener will do the job. Another great forearm exercise is using a short wooden dowel or metal bar with a rope tied to the middle and a weight plate or dumbbell tied to the other end of the rope, with some of the excess rope rolled several times around the dowel or bar. This is sometimes referred to as the *arm blaster* or *forearm roller*. You just hold the bar with the rope at full length and the weight resting on the ground, then with both arms extended and parallel to the earth, start winding up that rope. Don't lower your arms, and try to roll up that weight plate to the top and then back down to the bottom. Trust me on this one, your forearms are going to start feeling the burn. Just rep it out to your heart's content.

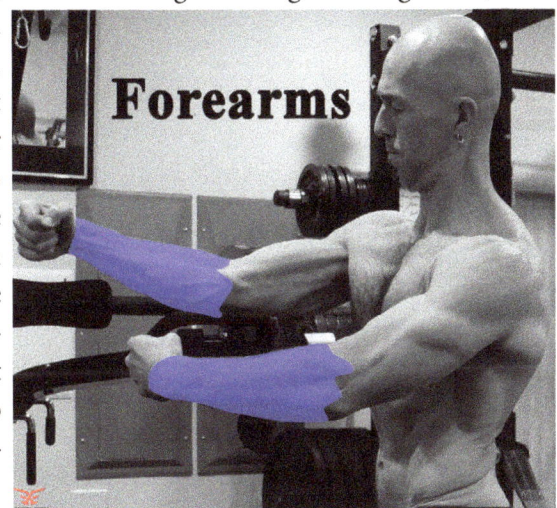

Shoulders

The shoulders are an interesting area of the body. The shoulder is a ball-and-socket joint, called the *glenohumeral joint*, composed of the head of the humorous and the scapula bones. Add the clavicle, and you've got what's called the shoulder girdle. The scapula, humerus, and clavicle together form a floating situation because the only bone-on-bone attachment to the body is where the clavicle meets the sternum. Instead, the shoulder girdle floats on a bed of underlying muscles, tendons, and ligaments.

The shoulder is one of the most mobile joints in the body. For this reason, it is easily injured. As we get older, we can lose the ability to raise our arms overhead, a movement that requires proper shoulder strength. That's why it is crucial to maintain shoulder stability and muscle balance through weight training exercises, stretching, and good body mechanics.

EXERLEAN: Resolution for the physique transformation of a lifetime.

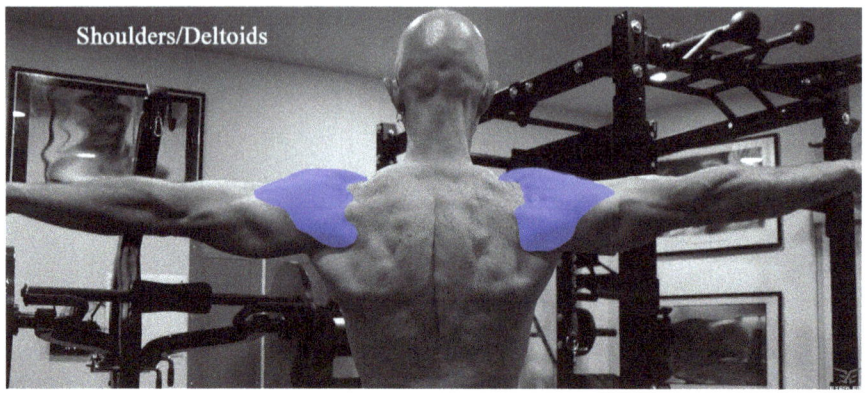

The shoulders are what gives a person's aesthetics or physique that broad, powerful look. For weight training purposes, the shoulders are composed of several muscles: the rotator cuff, the trapezius (traps), and the three heads of the deltoid (delts). These muscles mobilize the shoulder girdle, which includes the shoulder joint up the trapezius to the base of the neck, the shoulder area of the scapular muscles, and the uppermost area of the chest running down the clavicle to the sternum. For the EXERLEAN shoulder workout, we will leave out the upper chest since we'll focus on it separately. The rotator cuff will get strengthened coincidently by training the deltoids, chest, traps, arms, and back. (If you are having chronic shoulder pain, it could be due to an injury or muscle imbalance. It is wise to seek the advice of your doctor and request a referral or prescription for occupational or physical therapy to *evaluate and treat*.)

The shoulders are responsible for stability during any functional activity, resisted or unresisted, that involves the hands being moved away from the body by reaching, pressing, raising, pulling back, or swinging forward. An archer pulling the string back on a bow and arrow requires the stability of both shoulders simultaneously—one shoulder is pulling back, and the other is reaching out and extending. When you reach up to put a glass in the cupboard or wash your hair, this is primarily the work of your shoulders. A drywall installer must have strong and stable shoulders to press a sheet of rock up to the ceiling with one hand while the other grasps a drill and drives a screw into the drywall, securing it to the wood framing above.

There is a saying therapists use, "proximal stability for distal mobility,"

Chapter 12: Weight Training

with proximal meaning closest to the body and distal meaning farthest. In the case of the drywall installer, proximal refers to the shoulders, and distal refers to the hand pressing the sheetrock up into the ceiling. Without proximal stability, you cannot have distal mobility. This saying is usually referencing the necessity to have stability in the shoulders, spine, pelvis and hips in order to be able to manipulate the environment with our hands and feet.

A bodybuilder showcases their shoulders in one of the mandatory poses "back double arm biceps." With their back to the audience and head turned to the side, they curl both arms up and flex. It's an arm pose, but this is where deltoid development and aesthetics of the shoulder really pull it all together.

Chest

A rooster puffs up its chest to show a sign of force, to look bigger and badder. The chest is like the hood ornament on a car poised out in front of the body. What kind of car are you driving?

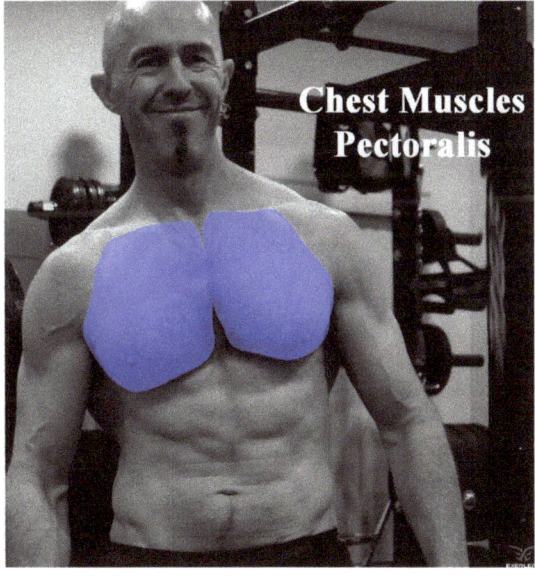

Regardless of the status of your chest now, we need to exercise it, and weight training will lead to a leaner, stronger, and well-shaped chest. Weight training will help you transform your hood ornament from a Yugo to a Ferrari.

The chest is composed of the upper, middle, and lower pectoral muscles (pecs). The pectorals spread from the base of the neck, below the clavicles down the rib cage to the bottom of the sternum and across the lower rib cage, then angle up to the armpits and shoulders.

Men and women both have pectoral or chest muscles, and both can have breasts with nipples on top of the chest muscles, often referred to as *man boobs* for men. Boobs or breasts cannot be worked out because they do not have muscles. They are either a female organ made up of the mammary glands and nipples whose function is to produce milk and feed baby humans after pregnancy, or, in the case of man boobs, a male feature composed of mostly excess body fat and nonfunctional nipples. In normal circumstances, men do not produce milk and cannot breastfeed.

We must also face the simple truth—the chest is a primary area of sexual attraction regardless of your gender. We can improve this attraction by improving the shape, symmetry, and aesthetics of the chest area. You can change your chest shape by developing the pectoral muscles underneath breasts or boobs. Women and men can do this by burning off the excess body fat around the breasts; in the case of man boobs, it will reveal a well-chiseled and masculine chest.

The chest is responsible for pushing or pressing things away from the body, namely by pushing the hands away from your body's core or resisting the drop back to your core. The primary driver in a boxer's punch is the chest muscle as it contracts and drives to extend the arm and then fist into the opponent's face. Pushing your body up from the floor during push-ups is a chest exercise. So is slamming the stick shift forward when driving a manual transmission or slapping someone's face. A football lineman needs a strong chest to push opponents away or drive them back.

A mandatory pose in bodybuilding competition is the "side chest," where the bodybuilder stands tall and sideways to the crowd, hands clasped with outside arm flexed and backside arm popping the shoulder forward to broadly display the pecs.

Abdominals

Over my last twenty-five years of training, the number one body part men and women ask me about is the abdominals, or abs. Everybody says, "I want to see my abs. How can I get a six-pack like the fitness people on Instagram?"

Abs are like the beautiful grill on the front of a car, the face of the human body, and a symbol of athletic prestige. A healthy-looking gut is attractive; it's sex appeal at its best.

When humans are on the lookout for a mate, we are instinctually drawn in by physical aspects, then personality. That's why it is natural to avoid someone with an obese belly, beer belly, or keg gut. Can you say heart attack, stroke, and early death? Research proves that your waist measurement and the shape of your belly—which blankets your abdominal muscles—is a key predictor or measure of your general health or "unhealth."

So what exactly do the abdominals do? If you are lying down and want to get up, you need abdominals to flex and elevate your upper body so your hand can grasp something and pull, then engage your legs to stand. That's why abdominals are a main contributor to getting in and out of bed. Have you ever seen a person struggling with this? I see it in the hospital every day with people who are 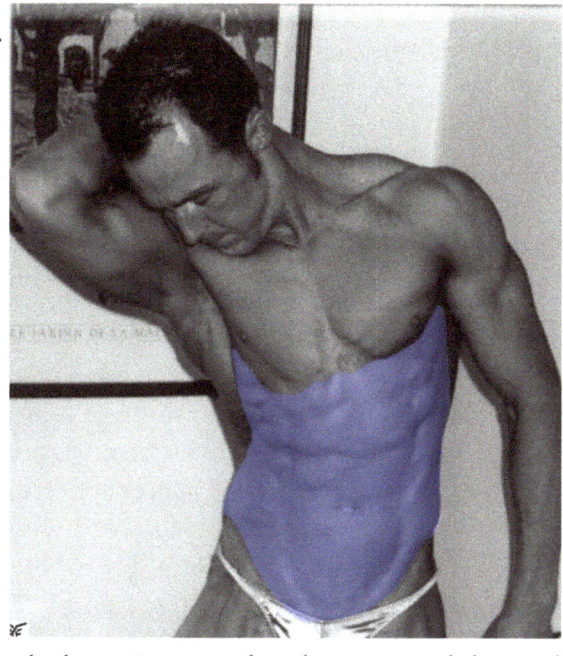 severely deconditioned and obese. Because they have poor abdominal strength, they use momentum to jerk themselves left, then right to heave themselves off their backs and over the edge of the bed. A downhill skier uses their abdominals every time they turn left to right or right to left, or when they bounce in and out of moguls.

A common misconception is that to see your abs, you need to do many reps of abs exercises or use a special abs machine. This is pure marketing from years of exposure to commercials and ads. Those gimmicky exercise devices may help you get a good abs workout, but they have jack shit to do with helping you see your abs or attain a six-pack.

Please burn this into your memory: **If you want to see the muscular details of your abs or any other muscle in your body, then the only way to achieve that goal is by removing the body fat covering them up.** This can be achieved only through your diet and body fat incineration through the metabolic pathway. You can do a zillion reps of abdominal exercises to make your abs stronger and better developed, but it won't remove the fat that is hiding them from view.

At first, nearly every client I encounter believes that if they do sit-ups, leg lifts, and crunches or use that special workout device they saw on TV, they will get a six-pack. But everybody already has washboard abs. Every typical human is born with abs; our fat just obstructs them from view. In fact, I rarely did abs exercises during my younger days of bodybuilding competition, yet I always had one of the most shredded six-packs in the entire competition. This is because I mastered the art of fat burning and living lean.

Now that we have let that sink in, why should we even work out our abdominals?

Now that I am older and more mature, I have started to do abs once or twice a week to stabilize my core for injury prevention. As we get older, we become more prone to spine and other musculoskeletal injuries, strains, or sprains. To maintain a toned body and stability, we need to be in a constant state of condition so we can endure the occupational workloads of life. Because the abdominals are the main support muscles of the core or trunk of the human body, doing abs exercises keeps the abdominals toned and strong to help stabilize your body.

Other than the spine, the abdominals are the body's only core stabilizers, and the better conditioning they are in, the better your core strength. Core strength is important for injury prevention, specifically to the spine during work, exercise, and leisure activities; trunk control; and proper posture of the human body. The abdominals also are the only protective layer between the outside environment and the fragile inner organs and guts. That's why a well-developed, strong set of abs can take a boxer's punch like a brick wall, while a weak and deconditioned set of abs will let that same punch push through to the guts and liver, smashing the spine. Ouch!

Having strong abs helps maintain core stability during heavy weight training like deadlifts, squats, and clean and jerks while helping prevent injury.

To sum it up, the goals of abdominal exercises is to gain and maintain core stability and strength to maximize our occupational performance during life's many activities, ranging from self-care to extreme athletics.

Chapter 12: Weight Training

At a minimum, we need to engage in abdominal exercises for injury prevention.

One of the mandatory poses in a bodybuilding competition is the "front abdominal thighs." The goal is to showcase a great set of abs and the striations of the obliques, the abs muscles on the sides of your core. It's typically delivered with both hands behind the head and contracting the elbows toward the audience, then leaning into and squeezing the obliques, with the outside leg flexing and toes extended to the ground. Bodybuilders be like, "Boom, check out these babies," leaving the jaw-dropping audience wanting to go home and do some abs exercises.

Back

The back is the bed of the body, the foundation for all gross, open, or large-extension movements. Extension is what keeps us standing erect. The muscles of the back control the spine and brace the shoulder girdle during work.

The back is one of the least talked about body parts. We always notice someone's nice abs, chest, or buttocks, but rarely do we hear people commenting about someone's back. Too bad because the back, when well developed and chiseled, showcases your power and strength. Power is a good thing. It's what determines your ability to move heavy objects.

A back can be attractive and sexy as well as powerful, so long as it is lean. A lean physique has well-defined shoulder

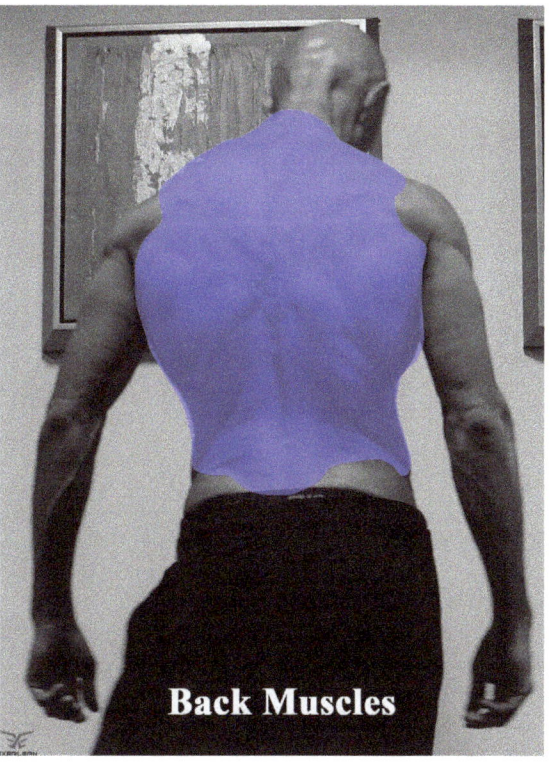

Back Muscles

blades, valleys, and hills between all the different muscles of the back. A fat back just looks like a big, flat smooth marshmallow with no defining attributes other than rolls, folds, or an innertube waist, depending on a person's level of obesity.

Rowing a boat, playing tug-of-war, and doing pull-ups all depend on the back muscles. When you pull a garbage sack liner out of the can, this is your upper back pulling it out. Therapists and nurses in the hospital setting get back injuries because they are always helping patients get out of bed, stand, and walk, which is all back musculature bracing the spine for this pulling work. Having a strong and conditioned back is key in injury prevention for any kind of lifting occupation or activity.

The "back lat spread" (*lat* is short for *latissimus*) is a mandatory pose during a bodybuilding competition. The bodybuilder's back faces the audience, with one leg slightly farther back, with toes extended flexing the calf and hamstrings, while both arms are flexed with thumbs hooking the waist and elbows popping forward to spread the back out as wide as possible.

A well-developed back is thick, with muscle from the spine out, and tapers from a broad upper back to a thin waist. Boom! Can you say hourglass figure dialed in? It doesn't matter if you're a man or woman, the hourglass shape is a healthy shape. Wide, keg-shaped, pear-shaped, and apple-shaped bodies are all an early death sentence, according to research.

So, let's change the shape of our body and work out our back! The most common back exercises include wide-grip pull-ups, deadlifts, and rows.

Legs

Legs are powerful and strong, like a tree's roots that lead up to the truck and stabilize the tree to the ground. A tree's roots are nearly equal in size to the branches that extend from the truck. For us, the trunk is our waistline, and the roots are our legs. For the legs, we include all muscles below the waist directly attached to the pelvis, femur, and tibia and fibula (shin and calf bones). The butt, or *gluteus maximus*, is the largest muscle in the human body.

The glute muscles: The glute muscles include the gluteus minimus, medius, and maximus. These are the most important muscles in the

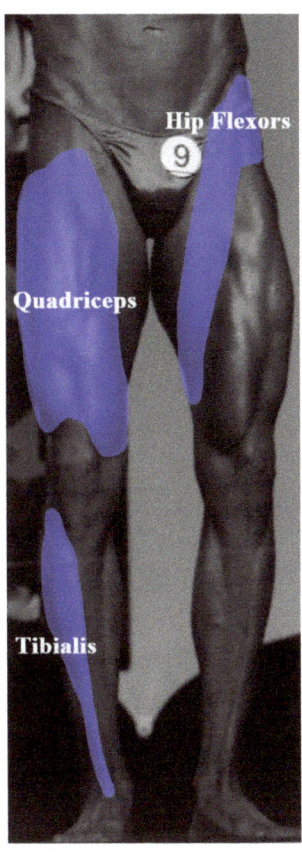

human body to keep us strong. They are the main contributor to being able to stand from a chair, get off the toilet, and squat down to the ground to pick something up. Everybody thinks these jobs are all quads, but this is not the case. The glutes and hamstrings are what allows us to bend down and pick something up while keeping our legs straight. The quads aid in the low squat and are primary in kicking a ball. The calf muscles allow us to stand on our toes to reach up high in a cupboard. The glutes do the driving.

The legs are the key to our mobility. They allow us to walk, jog, run, climb, and descend our environment. Without legs, we have to rely on our arms and in most cases a wheelchair or scooter.

Weight training the legs leads to improved muscle mass, strength, and function. A leg workout is a great fat-burning workout as well because of the amount of energy leg exercises require. Going up and down stairs is a great leg exercise. Climbing uphill and downhill, especially with a backpack on, is a great way to train your legs. These activities stimulate muscle strengthening in the legs because of added resistance from the environment—that is, the added personal gear. The legs will not get stronger or build muscle tissue without a high level of sustained resistance. Achieving the legs of a professional or competitive athlete requires such a high degree of resistance to stimulate them to change that in my experience, it is necessary to go to a gym or have gym equipment at home to achieve a successful workout.

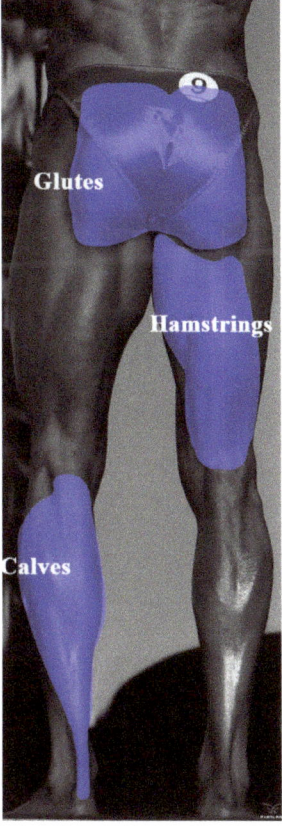

The most common exercises include squats, deadlifts, straight-leg deadlifts, lunges, leg presses, and heel raises.

A mandatory pose in a bodybuilding competition is the "most muscular pose." This pose involves hands on the upper buttocks/outer hip area and elbows popped toward the crowd while flexing the arms, chest, abs, and legs. The upper body is usually the main show at a competition, but the legs are the foundation that pulls the entire physique together.

A great set of legs is sexy. For women, long and toned legs with good musculature are considered attractive and healthy. For men, well-developed muscular legs with bigger calves are viewed as masculine and powerful. For both sexes, well-developed and muscular glutes are considered sexy, attractive, and healthy. It's no lie that when someone is in great physical health, their legs and butt look great in a pair of jeans. This is subjective, of course, but good legs and a good butt is well marketed and has been upheld as ideal by the majority of people on earth for the history of humankind. Most clothing companies don't use obese or morbidly obese male or female models for their clothing, and they shouldn't. When they do, ask yourself: Is this an advertisement of a healthy person? A role model, a physique to model myself by? Most people don't want to see an unhealthy body awkwardly displayed. This is confusing, and we must prevent society from accepting obesity as okay or, worse yet, desirable. It's like advertising a set of jeans using a model smoking a cigarette. TV and radio advertising with smoking has actually been against the law in the United States since 1971.

Timing for Your Weight Training Program

So, we have broken down the body into six major groups: arms, chest, shoulders, back, abdominals, and legs. Now that you know what to work out, it's time to start lifting weights and physically change things for the better!

There are different methods, protocols, programs, and styles of weight training. Breaking down the body into groups is a great method to get the whole body worked out over a week without leaving anything out. This is a typical muscle split routine or program. You can split your muscles into any arrangement you want. Some people like to do arms alone, or arms and shoulders, or arms plus shoulders and chest. Other people like to break the body into upper body and lower body. You can also do individual muscle workouts if you want, like a biceps workout where you do many different biceps exercises in varying reps, sets, and speeds to really nail 'em. Sometimes it is necessary to do a whole-body workout to make sure you are getting all your muscles in during the week, especially if you are crunched for time.

Timing of your weight training workout will make a difference in the outcome. First, I want to get one thing clear: the most important thing about weight training regardless of timing, format, or duration is that you actually do it. Action counts. Skipping weight training leads to slower progress and less results over time.

From here on out, let's refer to "weight training" as your "workout" and "cardiovascular training" as "cardio." These are the typical meanings in fitness or bodybuilding jargon. That being said, timing—or the time of day you complete your workout—produces different benefits. If you do your weight training first thing in the morning, you'll capture the body in a state of full rejuvenation, of full strength, and primed for work: ready to rock and roll. An early morning workout on an empty stomach can result in fat burning as well as muscle training. A negative side effect of this is that you will lose your animal strength and fatigue much quicker during your workout than you would later in the day with calories on board. If you decide to do your weight training session in the morning, I recommend having a protein shake or something prior to your workout.

I went from doing my workouts every day after work in the late afternoons to every morning at 4:00 a.m. in college. I was able to maintain my physique and strength through all the years of studying and homework. Still, I prefer to do an after-work workout (late afternoon) versus a before-work workout; the later a weight training session, the stronger and more prepared the body is to engage an onslaught of damage. Cardio, on the other hand, achieves the best results on an empty stomach first thing in the morning. I refer to this as *fasted cardio*. I've dedicated an entire chapter to this.

Picture your body like a sponge. Over the course of a day, you eat meals, drink shakes, take vitamins and supplements, and warm up all the body parts. Your sponge is full and ready for anything. Then by the end of the day, after completing all your work, your sponge becomes empty again and needs to rest and recover. A workout that takes place later in the day with a full sponge will give you fuller, harder, and stronger muscles, which makes heavier lifting easier as well as improves your muscle endurance, ensuring you'll make it through all the preplanned sets and reps. The night after a workout, your body uses any remaining nutrients and residual calories in the digestive tract as well as pulls from the body's storage areas to use for cellular repair, muscle synthesis, and chemical replenishment. By morning, your sponge is empty again. Working out on an empty sponge means engaging in exercises with empty muscles, low or no calories from food, and cold body parts. Morning workouts require sufficient warm-ups and stretching, increased mental discipline and fortitude. Man, but let me tell you! A successful early morning workout session leaves you cocked, locked, and ready to rock for the remainder of the day. You'll be fully pumped up and warmed up, and you will have awoken the body in a warrior fashion. The empty-sponge body is now primed to absorb anything calorie-wise for recovery and to prepare for the next barrage of lift-rest-repeat.

Back in the day I purchased a workout program called Shock Treatment, which came with a weight training book, VHS, and nutritional supplement. Shock Treatment was all about doing sets of one hundred repetitions per exercise. Can you say ouch? Talk about delayed onset muscle soreness, or DOMS for short. One hundred repetitions per set should be reserved for the seasoned athlete; you must work up to this level of training before taking on the endeavor. I refer to DOMS as EXERPAIN because it is exercise-induced pain and post-workout residual pain that remains during the next few days of healing. EXERPAIN is good pain.

Shock Treatment is a workout format designed by Joe Weider, the father of bodybuilding, to help bodybuilders break out of a plateau or just get a killer workout in. EXERPAIN is my own version of a shock treatment–type workout program. I designed EXERPAIN to bust anybody out of an exercise plateau—CrossFit, bodybuilding, fitness, powerlifting, or any fashion of athletic performance. EXERPAIN will be released in late 2023.

For now, there are many workout programs out there. Anyone can design or come up with their own workout routine that works best for them. Some make sense and are effective; some are a waste of time. It all depends on your knowledge and experience. Many programs have been designed to achieve specific results. Sometimes it is necessary to move to a different program, especially if the one you are familiar with isn't producing positive results or gains. Many people will switch workout styles every so often just to keep the body guessing, to prevent plateaus, or to promote new gains. The body responds well to variation in workouts.

I recommend switching things up when you notice you aren't getting stronger after a few weeks. You don't have to change workout programs, though. Other ways you can add variety or surprise the body is to change the reps and sets, add in drop sets, or go past failure. *Drop sets* are when you do repetitions to failure or muscle fatigue, then drop to a lower weight and do more reps during the same set. Then drop it again and do more reps, and so on until you just can't take the pain or lift with proper form anymore. Drop sets are a great method to damage the muscle tissues to achieve strength and muscle gains. Going *past failure* is when your spotter begins assisting you to get more reps after you reach failure. This technique will totally annihilate the muscles being worked because you are not dropping the weight to a lower weight but continuing to engage your body at the same weight for more reps. This is an awesome method to get stronger fast.

There is no real way to know which format, program, or timing will work best for you until you try a bunch, compare how you feel, and look at the results you achieved or didn't achieve. Do you have to follow a program to get positive results? No. Will it get you better results? Most likely. Remember, what is most important is that you are working against resistance. Picking shit up and putting it back down, pushing it forward or pulling it back, pushing it up or pulling it down. Whatever it takes so long as you're tearing down muscles so they will build back up during rest and recovery. As far as I'm concerned, if you are engaging in any workout at all on a weekly basis, then you are doing what is necessary for EXERLEAN. You can always change things up or home in on symmetry, focus areas, or another workout format after you become comfortable in your own skin.

As long as you are working out, you're on the path to win! I have designed a specialized workout program called Chaining, a "designer" workout because it was specifically designed by me to transform the human body through exercise and weight training. So, what is Chaining, and how do you do it?

CHAPTER 13

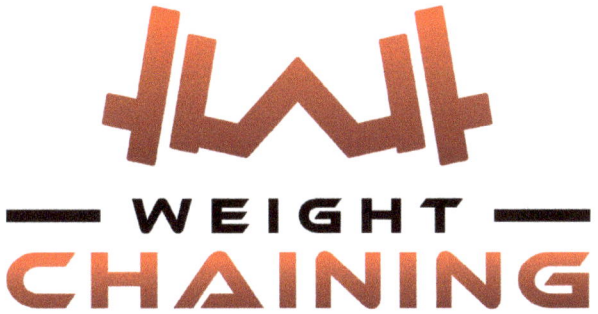

WEIGHT CHAINING

IN THE WORLD of weight training, there are a zillion different programs, formats, and styles. You can do high reps, low reps, one set, two sets, three sets, or more, drop sets, past failure, instinctive, upper body, lower body, or splits, plus a plethora of other options.

People typically experiment with a different number of sets and reps to figure out what gets their body to respond best. There are so many different exercises to do for each muscle or body part, and one may feel better than another, work better, or achieve better results. You've just gotta put in enough reps and sets over time to figure out how your body responds best and what exercises achieve positive results for you.

In my experience, there are preferred workout formats and protocols. Some exercises work better than others. A designer workout program can work well for one person but not for the next for multiple reasons. In my expert opinion, some workout formats achieve better results than others. Some workout programs are better because they are faster or require fewer workouts. Sometimes a program is better purely because it fits into your lifestyle and schedule better than another. Some workout formats and programs get better results than others because the best exercises are incorporated. You'll just have to experiment and put in the necessary time to figure it all out.

Down the road, after you have mastered your body and your exercise routine, you can modify your workout, add to it, or try something new you've been interested in. For now, I want to help you get started with a designer workout protocol I invented. The goal is to get every muscle worked at least once a week, in as few as two days a week, in a way that promotes extension, fall prevention, strengthening, fat burning, and muscle development.

The designer workout program I am talking about is called *Chaining*. Weight training becomes *weight chaining*. I have included the basics of the Chaining program in this book to give you a great workout protocol and to help you kick-start your transformation. I also have written a separate book specifically for the Chaining workout program that goes in detail on the three different phases of the Chaining program, its variations, and other strategic body-altering processes.

I recommend phase one of the Weight Chaining format in your EXERLEAN healthstyle transformation. It is low impact, gets all your muscles in, and can be done in two workouts a week. This format will help keep you from becoming overwhelmed, burnt out, and overtrained.

Before I show you how to do the workout, you need to know more about the muscles involved. The muscles of the human body can be divided into two parts: the *anterior chain* and the *posterior chain*.

Anterior: The front side

Posterior: The backside

The anterior chain refers to the muscles on the front of your body that contribute to your body curling up into a ball, otherwise known as *flexion*.

The posterior chain refers to all the muscles on the back of your body that extend all your appendages out and away from your body and also keep you upright against the force of gravity, which is always pulling us down to the earth.

The anterior chain succumbs to the forces of gravity. The posterior chain fights against the forces of gravity to keep us upright.

The anterior chain is our defensive strategy. The anterior chain will contract to protect us from frontal assault, an assault by any force that could injure our bodies, like the steering wheel impact in a rear-end collision, a punch to the gut, or a fall to the ground. To protect us, our abdominals and chest contract, and our arms and legs curl in and brace the body for impact.

As we age, the posterior chain begins to succumb to the forces of gravity. As our bodies weaken with the aging process, we start to hunch over and shorten. You can fight against gravity and the negative effects of aging through strength training and conditioning of the anterior and posterior chains.

Chaining is different from the typical muscle splits that most people engage in for weight training and strengthening. Typical muscle split training does not focus on function but on individual body parts and their muscle contractions separate from the body as a whole. Focusing on each body part individually is not bad—in fact, it is the typical method we are trained to engage in. We learn young to train body parts—chest, arms, legs, shoulders, abs, calves, and back. We are trained in sports and athletic training to focus on working body parts or a combination of body parts.

Chaining works individual muscles and their muscle synergies, specifically flexion and the extension of the human body as a whole. Muscle synergies refers to a group of muscles that act together to achieve a functional outcome based on one neural command. For example, when a boxer throws a punch, the brain does not send separate signals to each individual muscle involved in the motion but rather one signal responsible for coactivating a "chain" of muscles that execute the punch in one rapid and fluid motion.

A muscle synergy can activate multiple muscles, or a single muscle can be part of multiple muscle synergies. The anterior and posterior chains are often involved cooperatively in many muscle synergies. Imagine a gymnast performing a backflip. The flip starts in extension of the posterior chain, then flexion of the anterior chain in one fluid movement that results in her landing on her feet. Chaining is "functional" weight training, as the goal is to maximize the function and performance of either chain, which improves posture, self-care, and mobility.

One of the benefits of Chaining is the convenience of getting all your muscles trained in two workouts versus three to six, which is common for many programs. Most of the time when figuring out how often to work out, we use a ratio of exercising muscles and time—that is, time needed for rest and recovery after a muscle or muscle group has been trained. A trained muscle or muscle group typically needs two to three days of rest and recovery before it can be trained again. Knowing this, the typical muscle split of three to six workouts only allows working out each muscle once a week, unless you decide to weight train every day without much rest. Chaining is a two-day split that incorporates all muscles. This allows you to hit each muscle twice a week with ease and still have three complete days of rest between workouts. This, in theory, makes it possible to achieve twice as much mass and strengthening gains. Now, that's efficient and productive if you ask me!

To keep things simple, it is sufficient to weight train each muscle or muscle group—anterior and posterior muscle groups, in our case—once a week. This is the typical or average training protocol for most people. Therefore, following the Chaining protocol will have you weight training two days a week. This gives you five days of rest and recovery. Remember, weight training is exercise but separate from cardio. Cardio can and should be performed daily until the end of days.

The Chaining protocol starts with the anterior chain and ends with the posterior chain. This means at the start of your program, the anterior chain will be completed on day one, then the posterior chain on the next workout within a day or two. The reason for this order is to promote extensor tone over flexion tone whenever your body is in a resting state. The muscles that increase tone at rest will always be the muscles that were last pumped up from a workout. Because posture depends on good posterior chain tone and conditioning, ending with the posterior chain workout will result in lasting extensor tone at rest. This promotes remaining upright in good posture and fighting against the forces of gravity, which we've said is especially beneficially as you age.

So let's say it's a new week. It's Monday, and we are going to work out. The first workout will be the anterior chain workout. The next workout, which should be on Tuesday or Wednesday, will be the posterior chain workout. After Monday's anterior chain workout, your body will tend toward flexion because of the increased resting tone of your anterior chain. The next workout day, your posterior chain workout will dominate over the resting tone of the anterior chain, which will promote extension of your body until next Monday's anterior chain workout.

The increased tone from weight training a muscle or muscle group decreases over time, so the next workout will have dominant tone over the muscles of the last workout purely due to being a younger workout. So although it's not necessary, the best scenario for Chaining is to do the posterior chain the day after the anterior chain without a day of rest.

Anterior Chain Muscles

Whether it is an anterior or posterior chain workout, I find that working from top to bottom or bottom up works best rather than jumping around, since it keeps the workout organized.

So, starting from the top down, the muscle groups we'll exercise in the anterior chain workout are:

1. Anterior deltoids
2. Biceps
3. Chest
4. Abdominals
5. Hip flexors
6. Quadriceps
7. Tibialis

The *anterior deltoids*, or delts, are the front side of your shoulders just above the biceps. The front delts are part of the function of picking things up, albeit more of a stabilizing muscle when arm curling. The deltoid is made up of three muscle bellies, otherwise called the heads of the deltoid. We will be working the middle and posterior delts along with the trapezius in the posterior chain workout.

The *biceps* muscles are responsible for the flexion of the arm, or bringing the hand closer to the body. As we mentioned in the last chapter, the biceps pull things toward the body and are considered the most popular "showcase" muscles.

The *chest* is a large, broad muscle that can be divided into three parts: upper, middle, and lower chest, each responsible for a separate direction of movement. The lower chest is used in dips or pushing the arms away from the body *down* to the ground. The middle chest is the main body of the chest and is responsible for pushing *straight out* and away from the body. It contributes to the function of the upper and lower chest. The upper chest is responsible for pushing things *up* in the air and away from the body, like in a bench press.

The *abdominals* connect the lower rib cage to the pelvis and extend from the center of your belly around to your back. The abdominals are responsible for holding the center, or core, of your body together. As we discussed previously, they are stabilizers in movement and protection for your inner guts and organs. The center of the abdominals, the rectus sheath, is responsible for trunk or core flexion, and when it's lean, it gives us the envied six-pack. The left and right sides of the rectus sheath are called the obliques, which move the body in flexion and sideways. The obliques look serrated and chiseled in a lean physique.

The *hip flexors* are not typically a focus in a workout, but they should be as they are a vital component of the anterior chain. The hip flexors are a small muscle group connecting your upper leg to your pelvis and function by flexing your leg toward your upper body, for example, when you bring your knee up when going up and down stairs, or when you are lying flat in bed and lift your legs up and over the edge of the bed—otherwise called *straight leg raises*.

The *quadriceps*, or quads, are the big muscle group in the front of your upper leg connecting your knee to your pelvis. The quads are responsible for standing up from a chair, going up stairs, kicking a ball, and getting off the toilet. The quads are a strong force and major contributor to mobility in general.

The *tibialis* is the long skinny muscle in the front of your lower leg connecting the lower knee to the top of the ankle. Like hip flexors, it's not typically focused on in a workout but should be as a vital component in the anterior chain. The tibialis moves your foot into dorsi-flexion—meaning it moves the end of your foot or toes up toward your body. When you walk, the tibialis is responsible for making sure you don't stub your toes into the ground or keeping the tips of the skis up when downhill skiing.

Chapter 13: Weight Chaining

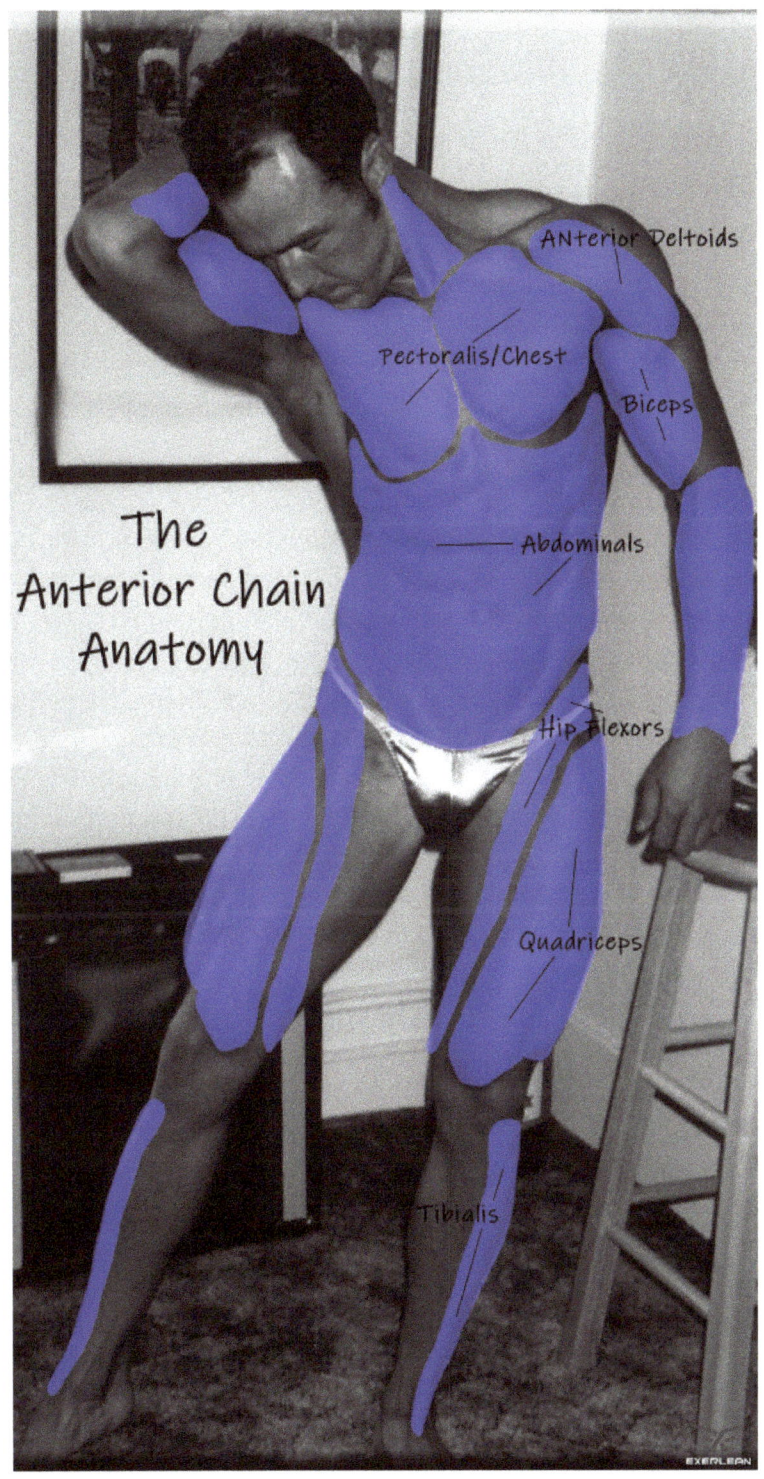

EXERLEAN 117

Posterior Chain Muscles

Here are the posterior chain muscles top to bottom:

1. Trapezius
2. Top/middle and rear/posterior deltoids
3. Triceps
4. Back
5. Lumbar
6. Glutes
7. Hamstrings
8. Calves

The *trapezius* is a very important and powerful diamond-shaped muscle unit spreading over the top and middle of the back muscles. The traps attach from the base of the back of the neck and spread out to each posterior shoulder, then make a V-shaped taper back down to the spine.

When looking directly at someone's front side, the traps are the muscle humps between the shoulders and the neck. Bodybuilders, power-lifters, and generally strong people have well-developed and pronounced traps. The traps are incorporated into many different muscle synergies of the shoulder and back. The main movement or function of the traps is shrugging, or lifting your shoulders toward your ears. The traps are also involved with rowing, pulling objects upward, or performing upper-back workloads. When you pick up something and carry it for a distance, the traps are hardworking stabilizers.

The *upper or middle and rear or posterior deltoids* are responsible for picking up your arms sideways and to the rear, moving your arms away from your body. These posterior chain muscles give our shoulders a narrow or wide stance depending on their development.

Toned and ready shoulders help maintain an erect and extended posture. Most people have forward protracted shoulders or falling shoulders, making them look hunched over. Well-developed and toned delts, traps, and back help keep our shoulders retracted and ready for action.

Triceps or tris are two-thirds of the upper-arm girth. This posterior chain muscle group takes up the whole backside of the arm from the shoulder to the elbow. The triceps are responsible for extending your elbow out to full open position, helping you stand out of a chair by pushing on the arm rests and extending. Since the triceps are the bulk of your upper arm mass, they need a little more training then the biceps.

The *back* is the core of the posterior chain. It pulls up the head, pulls in the shoulders, and keeps us erected above our legs. The back is composed of large and small muscle groups and can take quite a beating. Its muscles drape off your neck down your shoulder girdles to your low back, attaching to your pelvis. They also attach in the armpits and wrap around to your spine. The back has muscles that contract toward the spine and others that contract with the spine. It is the main contributor to rowing, pulling, and posture and is responsible for carrying the biggest loads of all arm-involved lifting, moving, and carrying objects in general.

The *lumbar* spine is the lowest portion of the back and an important hinge between the upper and lower body. The lumbar muscles attach at the low spine and wrap into the pelvis. This posterior chain link is secondarily trained with the back but needs its own exercise or two to focus on extending and hyperextending the spine. A well-conditioned and flexible lumbar musculature is poised for maximal injury resistance and supports the body during all antigravity movements (away from the ground).

The buttocks or *glutes* are the fulcrum in lower-leg extension. Kicking the leg back as far as possible, or hyperextension, is the job of the glutes. This posterior chain muscle group is also a major contributor in standing from a chair, squatting, and climbing uphill. The glutes attach at the top and sides of the pelvis to the uppermost portions of the posterior upper leg. The glutes are the most important muscle group of the lower body to weight train because they keep us upright.

If you haven't noticed, most people have a rounded, muscular buttocks when they are young, which tends to become flat or nonexistent in the aging process. From my hospital experience and observations, there is an epidemic of flat butts. Poor ability to squat or maintain dynamic standing balance is a major contributor to falls in the aging, so we must prevent this loss of muscle as we age. The older we get, the more vital it is to weight train and make sure the glutes are a top priority. Ha! And you thought working the booty was for the young. When you're young, the goal of booty training is sex appeal. The older you get, the goal shifts more to maintaining function.

The *hamstrings* are the large muscle group that runs from your buttocks to the back of your knee. This posterior chain muscle group is responsible for moving your foot toward your buttocks, or curling the lower leg. The hamstrings contribute to picking things up off the ground by stabilizing your legs during flexion of your upper torso at the hips. The hamstrings are considered the biceps of the legs.

The *calves* are the bottom of the posterior chain and often an overlooked muscle in a training program. The calves attach to the back of your knees and run down the back of your lower legs to the back of your ankle. The calves are an important muscle for standing on your toes when reaching up, climbing up stairs, climbing uphill, and performing all other mobility. As the "push-off" muscles in legs, they push off as we move our legs forward to make the next steps.

By working both the anterior and posterior chain muscle parts, the whole body is completed in two weight training workouts, leaving you with five days off to do other productive activities. And by completing the posterior chain a day or two after the anterior chain, you get an additional benefit of promoting extension of your body against gravity.

The anterior chain workout is usually shorter than the posterior chain because it has one less muscle group to exercise than the posterior chain. The posterior chain workout tends to consist of traditional powerlifting exercises, which also take longer to execute.

The more muscle bulk you have, the higher your resting metabolic rate. The higher your metabolism, the higher your fat-burning potential. The benefits of weight training are improved strength and power. Being strong and becoming more powerful is only a good thing! An additional benefit of weight training is muscle hypertrophy, which feels great and promotes increased muscle tone that is sustained long after a workout.

Welcome to the EXERLEAN Chain Gang.

Chapter 13: Weight Chaining

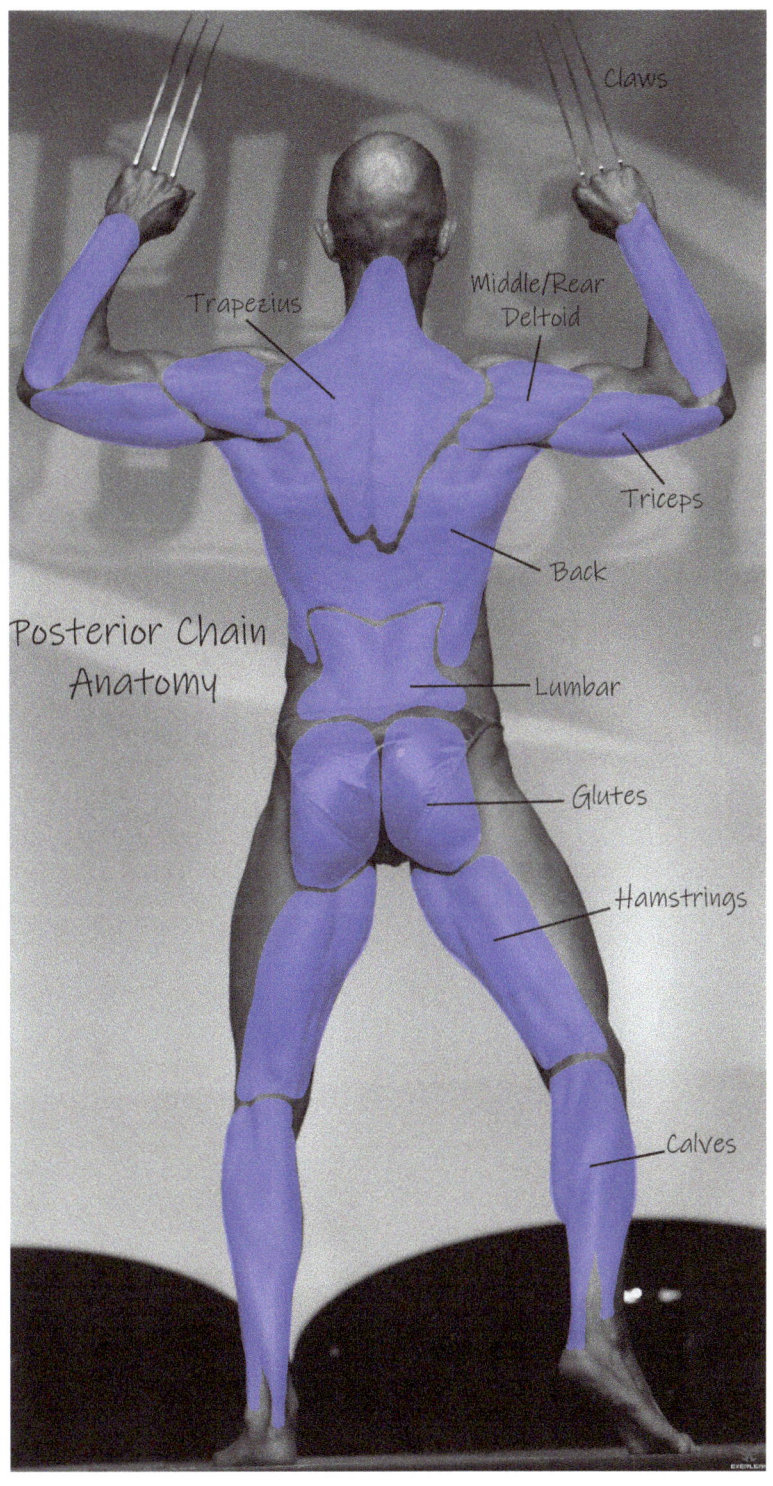

"Let's do this!"

When you finish reading this book, you will be ready to tackle your body transformation. You are gaining the know-how for change, and knowledge is power. Next you will learn about one of the greatest skills to burn off unwanted body fat. Fasted cardio: what is it and how you can take advantage of this transformational tool.

CHAPTER 14
Fasted Cardio

We've gone through the benefits of exercise, weight training, and the Weight Chaining protocol. Now let's move on to the ultimate fat-burning activity, fasted cardio.

First off, what is cardio?

Cardio is short for cardiovascular activity. *Cardiovascular* refers to the work of a beating heart and the resulting flow of blood through the bloodstream. The bloodstream is carrying vital nutrients and oxygen to the body for rejuvenation and energy. The faster your heart is beating, the more you are exerting. To increase your heart rate, you increase your exertion. Exertion is measured by the speed and intensity at which you are moving, the resistance settings on an exercise machine you're using, or the grade (incline) of the environment in which you are exercising. All can be adjusted to stimulate your heart rate to rise or fall.

Fasted refers to a state of burning calories from body fat instead of calories from food in your bloodstream, stomach, or gut. In this state, you are hungry and need to eat. You have low blood sugar and low gastrointestinal calorie deposits, so you are primed to pull from body fat stores to counteract your calorie deprivation.

Basically, to get into a fasted state, you need to deprive yourself of eating for a while.

Now, remember when we talked about catabolism, or #eatmuscles, in the principles of Bodinomics. Fasting, or starvation, eventually triggers a catabolic state in the body. Catabolism happens when the body is forced to start cannibalizing its own tissue for energy, either from body fat or muscle tissue. We want to cannibalize our body fat but *not* our muscle tissue.

To prevent the body from metabolizing muscle tissue for energy and promoting a state of *body fat* cannibalism specifically, we must carefully manipulate our body through macronutrient content and timing, also termed *macronutrient manipulation*. This is the secret to getting ripped like a bodybuilder. I will give you the full details on this secret science in chapter 20: The State. For now, I want to stay focused on the benefits of fasted cardio. Just remember that fasting is necessary to achieve the benefits of fasted cardio, and fasting correctly to get lean without losing lean body mass is described as "the State," a perfectly balanced state of sleep, wake, macronutrient consumption, carb depletion, and exercise timing that turns you into a body fat incinerator.

When you engage in fasted cardio, your body is primed to melt away body fat at the highest possible rate. I challenge you to engage in fasted cardio at any opportunity—in fact, make as many opportunities as you can for the rest of your life. Not only is fasted cardio your best weapon against obesity, it is also your best tool for maintaining a lean body composition. After you have achieved your desired body composition, you need to maintain your newly adopted healthstyle habits in the "maintenance phase" to sustain a healthy body and fitness conditioning for life.

The benefits of fasted cardio are plenty. Let's go through some of them now.

1. **Low blood sugar levels.** Low blood sugar promotes pulling energy from the adipose (fat) layer to use during work, exercise, or other activity.
2. **No food in the gut.** Without food in your system to use for energy, the body will pull from the adipose layer instead.
3. **Post-rested state.** When fasted cardio is executed first thing after sleeping, the body is rested and has rebalanced all body chemicals and hormones; therefore, it is ready for the day's activities.
4. **Increased endorphin release.** Cardiovascular exercise promotes the release of endorphins into the bloodstream to minimize pain and discomfort. These feel-good chemicals have lasting effects after exercise.

5. **Increased metabolism.** Engaging in fasted cardio turns up the body's metabolic threshold, which leads to increased calorie burning not only during exercise but for the rest of the day.
6. **Activation of cellular processes.** Fasted cardio promotes improved protein synthesis, meal absorption, and energy pathways in the body—that is, how your body converts nutrients into energy.
7. **Improved overall physiology.** Fasted cardio engages the heart, lungs, and other organs, leading to improved blood pressure, lower resting heart rate, improved respiratory function, maximum circulation, better skin, proper body water balance, and other body functions.
8. **Better sleep.** Fasted cardio completed first thing each day contributes to fatigue and exhaustion by the end of the day when it is time for bed. Aside from being easier to fall asleep, it improves your quality of restful sleep, or rapid eye movement (REM) sleep.
9. **Improved health and wellness.** In addition to better sleep, faster cardio improves your spirits, sense of well-being, self-confidence, and centeredness.
10. **Prevention of fat storage.** Fasted cardio boosts your metabolism from the get-go through the rest of your day. As we've mentioned, this is the best-case scenario for maintaining a lean, healthy body.

Now let's talk about timing. Like weight training, *when* you do fasting cardio determines whether you will receive the benefits of fasted cardio or just the benefits of regular nonfasted cardio. For cardio to become fasted cardio, there needs to be a period of at least *four hours since you last consumed calories* in any form, liquid or solid. This time frame is when you are in a restrictive diet and your body is deprived. According to the Mayo Clinic, digesting a meal takes six to eight hours for the food to be assimilated by the stomach and then the bowel, then eliminated.

This varies among individuals, for male or female, and by meal proportions and content.

Overall, the best time to perform fasted cardio is first thing in the morning after a full night's sleep, when your stomach and digestive tract are empty of calories, your muscle glycogen is at its lowest, and any energy the body will need to summate will be from your body fat stores. BOOM! Total body fat annihilation at its premium.

There is also a risk of burning up protein stores or muscle tissue during this catabolic or cannibalistic process. To preserve muscle tissue and promote fat burning during a workout or cardio, you can take amino acids and/or conjugated linoleic acid (CLA) supplements prior to your cardio. We'll talk about supplements more in the *LEAN* section of the book.

To fit fasted cardio into your day, you could wake up an hour earlier. Your last meal would be the evening before. Another way to fit it in is with an *after*-work fasted state. Let's say you are at work and eat your lunch at noon. To create a state of fasted cardio, you will avoid any calories after lunch and go jogging after work or head to the gym and put time in on an exercise machine, no sooner than 4:00 p.m. This small fast of at least four hours after lunch will be more of a fasted cardio benefit than if you ate your lunch at noon and did your cardio at 1:00 p.m., especially if lunch was lean and restricted. If your lunch was a total binge-out buffet or super calorie dense, then you can forget about "fasted" cardio for the rest of the day.

Fasted cardio is the number one *EXER* tool at your disposal to burn off body fat. Engaging in fasted cardio first thing in the morning will jack your metabolism and help you maintain a healthy body weight for life. With fasted cardio, you get the benefits of exercise and fat burning combined. Once a day for fifteen to forty-five minutes will suffice, and six to seven days a week is the goal.

How am I able to make this whole thing easier? By having an elliptical trainer at home. I wake up at 3:00 a.m. and do forty-five minutes on the elliptical, then write for an hour or work on another important goal. Then I get ready for my career job. Many successful people get up in the early darkness of the morning to capture this invaluable time of the day—basically, to get shit done that matters. When you get in the habit of early morning work, you'll find that this ends up being some of the most productive time of your day, with many mental and physical benefits. So, get up early and complete your fasted cardio!

CHAPTER 15
EXERPAIN

WHAT IS EXERPAIN? I conjured this portmanteau to clarify pain derived from undertaking any sort of exercise. It is my take on DOMS, delayed onset muscle soreness.

exercise + pain= EXERPAIN

EXERPAIN is also the name of my designer group exercise class based on EXERLEAN Chaining with the goal of shock and awe, set to release in 2021–2022. Stay tuned at exerlean.com. EXERPAIN is also my gamer tag in the world of video games, so if you're on Stream, Microsoft Live, Twitch, or EA, then you know it's me.

So why a chapter on EXERPAIN? Well, because pain is a major aspect of life in general, and exercise can lead to it, and should. That is, as long as you're doing it correctly. In my experience and from my observations, that delayed onset muscle soreness, or EXERPAIN, is the biggest culprit for people quitting on their hopes and dreams of getting in shape or losing weight. Post-exercise pain is what deconditioned and out-of-shape people experience after they start exercising to change their lives. (Heck, for them it can be painful exercising, too.)

Don't get me wrong here. Even the most experienced sports athletes, Olympians, and bodybuilders feel the effects of delayed onset muscle soreness. But the pain they feel is *nothing* compared to what a deconditioned nonexerciser feels. The morning after a nonexerciser hits it hard, they be crawlin' out of bed, draggin' themselves across the hall like a corpse zombie, trying to get to the bottle of painkillers in the kitchen.

It doesn't matter who you are; if you have not exercised in a long time, then you will have a high probability of experiencing higher-than-average amounts of EXERPAIN initially because you are so out of shape.

This is temporary!

EXERPAIN is pretty bad when you start out, but don't worry—if you stay consistent and keep moving forward, the intensity of EXERPAIN diminishes as you get in better shape. You can expect higher levels of EXERPAIN during the first two to three weeks of your weight training and exercise program, then your pain will start to lessen. As you get better conditioned to exercise, the post-exercise pain diminishes to the point that you have to train extra hard to achieve any sort of EXERPAIN. For a seasoned athlete or bodybuilder, this is a sign from the body that you did a good job. No more "oh, fuck me" pain. No more zombie movements or desperate searches for painkillers.

Push through.

Endure.

You can do this!

Most people quit exercise or weight training because of discomfort, pain, or fear. Don't quit! Stay with the program. Focus on your goals and do the work. The whole dang process gets easier week by week, and you want to be a *winner*. You control how you think and act, so think of EXERPAIN as good pain and your reward for killing it in the gym. Your badge of honor for doing what is necessary to change your life for the better. Your evidence of completing a great workout, one that's melting away your body fat. It's hard to imagine when you are a novice or beginner athlete, but trust me on this, successful athletes strive for EXERPAIN from getting in a great workout.

In addition to the DOMS you naturally experience after a vigorous weight training or cardiovascular workout, specific types of muscle contractions, called eccentric contractions, will lead to higher levels of DOMS than concentric contractions. An *eccentric contraction* is the slow release of a muscle fighting against resistance and relaxing toward the end range of motion—basically as far as it can safely extend. A *concentric contraction* is the type of tension from flexing a muscle and squeezing it hard, like flexing your biceps. The eccentric contraction for the biceps would be to slowly open the angle of your elbow from full biceps flexion (close to the body) to full extension, releasing slowly against resistance.

To get a brutal workout, many weightlifters will do slow-release *resisted* eccentric contractions, which cause a higher degree of muscle tissue damage and provoke a positive healing response.

The pain from DOMS occurs when skeletal muscle fiber and connective tissue (tendons, ligaments, and cartilage, which connect other tissues and organs) are damaged or break down from engaging in a repetitive strenuous workload. During exercise, the muscles work by withstanding a force or some other type of resistance. The heavier the resistance, the more muscle fibers are recruited, resulting in even more damage. The damaged muscle and connective tissue triggers a response from the body to transport blood and nutrients to the damaged area to repair and reinforce it, preparing it for the next onslaught of heavy work. This response also invokes a state of inflammation. Inflammation is likely the biggest contributor to pain itself. So, if you treat inflammation, you diminish pain.

It is pretty simple. The harder and longer manual labor or weightlifting is, the stronger and better conditioned the person. Keep in mind, though, that it is also important to avoid overtraining as this may result in a negative recovery process of muscle breakdown, fatigue, stress, and possibly injury.

There is a difference between the heavy work of manual labor and weight training. A long day at a manual labor job will not necessarily make your muscles bigger because the human body gets accustomed to daily work and will adapt to handle the repetitive stress. Your body will also condition and prepare itself only for that exact manual labor work, leaving many muscles unworked and neglected. Over time, this will result in muscle imbalances of strength and weakness in the body and can lead to chronic pain and body aches as we age.

Weight training focuses on the individual muscles or muscle groups, and focusing on them separately conditions them equally over time. Even people in manual labor jobs would benefit greatly, if not more so, from routine weight training to balance their body's muscle synergies, muscle strength, and muscle tone and readiness, as well as muscle development and physical aesthetics. They will improve performance and productivity and feel great at their job because they are trained and conditioned for the work to come.

Active and Passive Modalities: Treating EXERPAIN and Nonexercise-Related General Aches and Pain

Pain is a natural response from the body to make us aware of an injury or overstressed body area. The response should be rest, consuming protein and nutrients for healing, and participating in other activities that may promote or aid in healing. These other activities are referred to as treatment modalities, or modalities for short. Modalities are used to alleviate pain, promote circulation, decrease swelling or inflammation, calm muscle spasms or cramping, and in some cases, deliver medication to a specific area of the body.

Modalities are tools in your arsenal to treat pain, including EXERPAIN, by promoting healing and recovery. Modalities come in two forms, passive and active. Some examples of passive modalities are:

- Electrical muscle stimulation (e-stim or EMS)
- Ice packs
- Heat packs
- Oriental cupping
- Traction
- Joint mobilization
- Massage therapy
- Iontophoresis
- Kinesiology taping
- Acupuncture
- Light therapy
- Hypnosis
- Relaxation techniques
- Mindfulness
- Hydrotherapy, or hot tub (my favorite!)

Active modalities include:

- Exercise
- Stretching/warming up
- Mobility intervention

Strength training

Believe it or not, research shows that active therapy is far more beneficial and produces better long-term outcomes than passive modalities. In my opinion, this is because you can throw all the external forces you can muster at the human body, but none will have the power or efficacy of the body's internal processes for healing itself.

Passive modalities are exactly that, passive. They are delivered externally—on your body—and feel good at the time, and maybe for some time after. In the long run, though, most passive modalities deliver only temporary results.

Active modalities invoke an internal response in your body—actual physical healing or strengthening processes that lead to less pain when you're actively engaged and may be sustained long term. Engaging in active modalities can modify your body physically and affect other forces dealing with pain, such as improving your self-efficacy and diminishing your fear of avoiding the pain. Active modalities put the power in your hands. Passive modalities, however, can reinforce your feelings of powerlessness. They may lead to feelings of dependency and needing to return indefinitely to your healthcare provider, therapist, or doctor. How many people do you know who are addicted to going to the chiropractor or massage therapist and continue to complain about their pain?

Active modalities should always be the primary path to reducing pain and promoting healing. Passive modalities have their place and benefit, but they should only be used to support an active treatment plan. This will move you from a disempowering status to an empowering state of being.

Self-management and control is the goal. Remember, active modalities trigger internal body responses to treat pain.

Passive modalities are external stimuli that have less of an overall effect on long-term healing and pain than activity.

So, knowing all this, what do you do to help with the EXERPAIN? Well, you should take advantage of active modalities like stretching, warming up, and exercise to promote healing and reduce pain, and then add in any passive modalities you think will help you feel better, like soaking in a hot tub, applying ice packs, or using a foam roller. Just don't ever stop active therapy, and avoid getting caught in the cycle of passive therapy dependence. Any good PT, OT, chiropractor, or massage therapist will tell you this. It is more important for you to do the home programs they give you than the short sessions you have with them, which for the most part are just temporary fixes.

In my experience, the best results for alleviating general aches and pains is to engage in exercise that gets the blood circulating and warms up the body part that is hurting. Light cardio will warm up the entire body and increase blood flow, leading to less pain overall. For back pain, I have had the best results with consistent heavy weight training based on periodization. Periodization is using a prescribed or designed repetition, resistance, and timing regimen in order to prevent injury and over-training, as well as maximize strength building. A common periodized protocol is called *pyramid training*. Starting from the bottom of the pyramid with let's say twelve repetitions, then 10 repetitions on the next set, on down to the last set at the top of the pyramid, which is usually going for a 1RM/one-rep max. When I was young, I never had to warm up or stretch before a workout or manual labor, but now, if I don't warm up and stretch first, I'm almost certainly going to get a strain or injury. I like to hop on an elliptical trainer for about twelve minutes at a light to medium intensity to get my muscles and joints all warmed up and ready to rock. Before hitting the weights, I warm up my target muscles with a stretchy band.

I also find a few passive modalities helpful. Some that I routinely engage are:

1. **Hot tub.** I love getting in a hot tub for fifteen minutes in the evening. I have found the benefits of this type of heat therapy to be frickin' fantastic. It helps me relax before bed, relieves both physical and mental stress, decreases body aches and chronic pain, and improves my sleep.
2. **Massage therapy.** Research has found many benefits of massage, including treating muscle spasms, body aches, fibromyalgia, headaches, sports injuries, and myofascial pain. Other than the possible physical benefits of massage therapy, there are the obvious benefits of feeling fantastic, which often produces feelings of caring, comfort, and connection. Massage therapy can help you decrease or manage anxiety, stress, and emotional turmoil. I see a massage

therapist for deep tissue massage when the muscle tone in my back gets out of whack and needs a reset.

3. **Cold therapy.** In most cases, ice is the best treatment for a strain, sprain, bruising, or trauma that is causing inflammation or swelling. Ice, otherwise referred to as *cold therapy* or *cryotherapy*, works in the acute injury phase (within forty-eight hours of trauma or injury). It does this by slowing down the blood flow to the traumatized area of the body, therefore reducing inflammation and swelling. Cold therapy can also reduce nerve sensitivity, which diminishes pain. Remember, treat inflammation, eliminate pain.

Most people engage in passive modalities because they are easier, feel better, and can have powerful actual or placebo effects on our bodies and minds. Regardless, you should always use active modalities like stretching, pre-workout warm-ups, and exercise over passive modalities like massage, ice, or heat therapy. This results in you taking control away from someone else and giving it back to yourself. *Active* means you are in the driver's seat, which builds self-confidence, self-esteem, and success. Once you have control over your active self, you can add in passive modalities as support for the active, capturing the overall benefits of all the tools in your arsenal for healing and treating EXERPAIN!

PART 3
The "LEAN" in EXERLEAN

CHAPTER 16
Bodinomics: Nutrition

BEFORE WE MOVE into the how-tos of dieting, we need to establish a firm foundation of the *basics of nutrition* and the *science* on how the human body deals with food. This information is meant to be valuable for every person at any stage in life, from zero knowledge on nutrition to an experienced and successful bodybuilder. I state "bodybuilder," not "nutritionist" or "doctor," because I want you to have a different perspective—that of a seasoned bodybuilder—than that of the status quo. A warrior in the trenches knows the ins and outs of dieting. This information is delivered in a way that will help you achieve **real results**. I want to help you lose all that extra body fat at the fastest clip possible so you don't waste your life working on a program that will achieve lackluster results.

Many nutritionists and doctors I have dealt with are stuck in a mindset they were taught in college that is based around the U.S. government's *recommended daily allowance* (RDA). The RDA, in general, will help the average healthy person establish a basic healthy eating pattern based on calories and macronutrient ratios, but it will *not* help you lose body fat. There are trainers, therapists, doctors, and nutritionists out there who do know how to help you work out and burn body fat, but I implore you to let their physical status guide you. Are they obese?

When it comes to achieving weight loss or incinerating body fat, do *not* follow advice from someone who obviously does not follow their own advice or is unsuccessful with it.

Consider this: Would you invest your money with a rich person or a poor person? Likewise, don't waste your time or money investing in people who cannot help you.

This book is directed toward people without medical complications, diseases, or disabilities. Don't get me wrong—the knowledge and materials laid forth in this book will work for most people. If you are diabetic, disabled, or have some other form of disease or health predicament, then you are in special circumstances and should seek expert consultation and clearance from your doctor before beginning an exercise or dieting regime. If your doctor says that exercise, dieting, or weight loss won't benefit you, please get a second opinion. Only in rare circumstances is exercise or weight loss harmful to one's overall health and quest for longevity and wellness.

I want you to look honestly at yourself and your size, shape, weight, strength, flexibility, and function. If you feel like shit, look like shit, move like shit, and have shit for strength, then something or many things you are doing are causing this shitstorm in your life.

I am preparing you to take your health and wellness into your own hands. These unlocked secret strategies will help you take control of your body and do what is necessary to achieve a lean and strong body, and with it, the mind and soul will follow.

After you've achieved your weight loss goals, maintaining this healthy state of being is your lifelong plan.

No more yo-yo dieting. No more repetitive failures. Bye-bye body fat forever.

People fail at losing weight because they lack the knowledge, skill, and perseverance necessary for successful fat burning, particularly when it comes to diet. You need to learn the basic knowledge of human physiology and the science of nutrition, otherwise you will not fully understand the dieting, macronutrient manipulation, cycling, and fasting that we will be talking about. I've cut out all the shit that doesn't matter and laid out, in layman's terms, the stuff that does.

Food is what you eat. You take a bite, chew it up, and swallow it into your belly. Once the food is in your belly, you do not have control over what your body does with it. We do, however, know what is supposed to happen based on science and human physiology. Since we know what is supposed to happen in the human body in response to food, we can manipulate the response by strategically controlling what goes in. You control what goes into your belly though eating, and what you put in your mouth will have an indirect impact on what your body will do with it and the overall outcomes dealing with body composition, energy, and sleep.

Like the old saying goes, you are what you eat:

1. If you eat *protein*, then you are *muscle*.
2. If you eat *carbohydrates*, then you are *energized*.
3. If you eat *fat*, then you are *fat*.

What you choose to eat should complement your needs. If you are overweight or obese, then the last thing you need is fat or energy. You have enough stored in your skin's fat layer and should use that fuel before consuming more. If you are thin and weak, then you need to add more muscle mass to your frame by eating more protein and acquire more energy by consuming more carbohydrates. If you are in great shape already or have achieved a healthy, lean physique, then you need to maintain your awesomeness with a balance of fat, protein, and carbohydrates and calorie restriction.

What is food? Food is nutrients received from a mix of proteins, carbohydrates, fats, fiber, vitamins, minerals, and water. We get these nutrients from animals, fish, insects, trees, other plants, water, and supplementation. Basically, food is made up of smaller *macronutrients* (*macros* for short): proteins, carbohydrates, and fats. These macros have different and shared properties that benefit your body in some way. Each macro has calories and energy. Each macro has different values and a destined purpose in your body that will lead to predetermined outcomes. By strategically controlling the quantity, quality, and proportions of macros, you can externally influence what happens internally. You can take an *active* role through intake, which indirectly controls what happens *passively* inside your body.

This idea is vital to remember, believe, and comprehend: you have 100 percent control of what you put into your body.

What you put into your body, by choice, has an outcome that will be either positive or negative.

You are the boss, the CEO, the master controller of your body, and you must accept all responsibility for the results, good or bad. With the help of this program and through trial and error, you will learn how to earn positive results and steer away from negative outcomes.

Aside from water, vitamins, and minerals, the macros—the big three—are the main influences on your body composition and energy. We do not need to focus on vitamins and minerals because these are contained in the proteins, carbohydrates, and fats we consume.

Protein

Protein is the building block of the human body. **A gram of protein contains 4 calories.** So, for example, 40 grams of protein equals 160 calories. Protein has minimal if any influence on insulin release, so it doesn't affect your blood sugar levels. Remember, insulin is a deal breaker when it comes to weight loss; to burn more body fat, you must minimize or prevent insulin release.

Protein is the primary macro the body uses to create new muscle tissue, repair damaged tissue, and support brain function. Proteins also make up organs, antibodies, enzymes, and some hormones. So think of protein as your healer, constructor, and maintainer of wellness.

Protein is king.

There are up to one million different proteins in the body. They are made up of chains of amino acids. Amino acids are the building blocks of protein, and twenty amino acids make up all proteins. The human body can synthesize thirteen of these amino acids, and the other seven must come from foods we eat. These seven are called *essential amino acids*. It can be beneficial to supplement amino acids: for one, to make sure your body is getting all the essentials in, and two, to capture the muscle-preserving properties of amino acid supplementation during fasting and exercise. We will talk more in depth on amino acid supplementation in chapter 21.

Good-quality protein comes from beef, chicken, fish, wild game, pork, other animal meats, eggs, milk, protein powders, and amino acid supplementation. Many people are unaware that proteins are not created equal; in fact, there are very high quality and very low quality proteins. How do you know the quality of a protein source? The answer is the biological value scale (BV). We will talk more about the BV scale and determining the best quality proteins in an upcoming chapter.

Trimmed down to the simplest yet necessary elements, protein:

1. Is responsible for healing, repair, brain function, and maintaining and synthesizing new muscle fibers. Protein and the amino acids that make them up are considered the building blocks of the human body.
2. Has a caloric value of 4 calories for 1 gram.
3. Has a minimal effect on blood sugar levels and minimal if any effect on insulin response in the body.
4. Can be broken down into amino acids, which the body can reconstruct into the proteins it needs for repairing, building, or performing other functions.

Carbohydrates

Carbohydrates are energy. They provide fuel for the brain and body. Carbohydrates exist in three major forms: simple sugars, complex carbohydrates, and fibrous carbohydrates. Just like protein, **carbohydrates contain 4 calories per gram**. Carbohydrates are converted into glucose, the body's basic fuel. Carbohydrates are the main instigator of releasing insulin in the body in response to elevated blood sugar.

Carbohydrates are the bulk of the modern diet in most areas of the world and likely the number one contributor to the relentless surge in obesity rates. Think about it. If obesity is on a rising trend without signs of retreat, then maybe we need to look at the basics. What are people eating? Mostly carbs! Maybe people are eating too much carbs, or the wrong kinds of carbs, or both. We'll get to this solution in the coming chapters.

Simple Sugars

Simple sugars include the *oses*—sucrose, fructose, glucose, maltose, and lactose. These include table sugar (white sugar), brown sugar, beet sugar, milk sugar, any other sugar, honey, corn starch, and fructose and glucose from fruits and some vegetables. Some common sources of simple sugars are juicy fruits, pancake syrups, brown and table sugar condiments, frostings, desserts, candies and chocolates, jellies and jams, juice, soda pop, ice cream, and smoothies. Melons, berries, bananas, and juicy fruits like peaches, cherries, and plums are high in simple sugars. The sweet yummy and addictive tastes of nature come from simple sugars.

The release of insulin in the body is most affected by consuming simple sugars. The simpler the macronutrient molecule's structure, the easier it is for the digestive tract to break down. Simple sugars begin breaking down and assimilating with the body the moment they touch the tongue and interact with saliva. The faster a macronutrient is assimilated by the body, the more insulin the pancreas delivers. To prevent or minimize this release of insulin and boost fat burning, you should minimize simple sugars as much as possible.

The term *energy crash* refers to the rapid rise and then depression of blood sugar, which leads to a heightened state of energy and alertness followed by a state of low energy, physical burnout, and mental lethargy. Avoid the rapid rise in blood sugar, and you'll avoid the energy crash that follows.

Complex Carbohydrates

Complex carbohydrates are bigger and more complex molecule structures then their carb sisters, simple sugars. There are a few different types of complex carbohydrates, including starchy carbs, fibrous carbs, and glycogen. Starches and fiber come from food and may be converted to glucose, which is stored in your liver and muscles as glycogen, an energy source for the body to use later. Common starchy carbs include any type of potatoes, yams, rice, oatmeal, whole grain pastas and breads, couscous, multigrain cereals, beans and lentils, pumpkin, and squash. These calorie-dense carbohydrates are the bulk of most modern diets and are correlated with obesity when overconsumed. They take longer for the body to break down and digest than simple carbs, so they release insulin over a longer period than simple sugars. Complex carbs are a preferred energy source for endurance sports, powerlifting, work, and manual labor because they are more difficult for the body to break down and therefore provide sustained energy. Beans are the best complex carbohydrate for *dieting* and performance. We'll get more into why soon.

Fibrous Carbohydrates

Fibrous carbs are low in calories, have great nutritional value, and provide energy. They won't make you fatter. In fact, they will help you maintain weight or become thinner, so you can eat as much of these as you want. Fibrous carbohydrates include leafy greens, herbs, and vegetables like lettuce, cauliflower, peas, carrots, corn, broccoli, onions, cabbage, peppers, cucumbers, tomatoes, green beans, asparagus, and mushrooms (technically a fungus, but hey, they're on a salad).

Many complex carbohydrates like yams and potatoes are vegetables in the form of tubers. Please do not get caught up in the never-ending debate on what is and is not a vegetable or a fruit. This is a waste of your time.

Instead, focus on whether the carb is simple, complex, or fibrous. We are going to categorize based on these, not on whether the food is a fruit, vegetable, or other. In the end, all that matters is the reaction the food has in your body.

Here is a quick summary of the three types of carbohydrates:

1. **Simple carbohydrates.** These are high calorie, blood sugar spiking, insulin triggering, rapid energy spiking with equally rapid burnout, brain fueling, and highly addictive.
2. **Complex carbohydrates.** These are high calorie, calorie dense, mild to moderate blood sugar spiking, insulin triggering, slow releasing for sustainable energy, brain fueling, and moderately addictive.
3. **Fibrous carbohydrates.** Fibers are low calorie, calorie thin, zero to mild blood sugar spiking, low to no insulin triggering, full of nutrients that promote energy and brain health, and low addictive.

Trimmed down to the simplest yet necessary elements, carbohydrates:

1. Are responsible for providing energy for the body to use for life, work, and brain function.
2. Have a caloric value of 4 calories for 1 gram.

3. Raise blood sugar levels in the body and are the primary factor in triggering an insulin response.
4. Are broken down into glucose, which the body uses for energy, glycogen replenishment, and other body functions.

Just like the quality of protein can be measured with the BV scale, carbohydrates can be measured or scored using the glycemic index, or GI, scale. The BV and GI scales will be important tools in your journey toward body fat incineration. We'll get into the GI scale soon.

Fats

Also called lipids, fats are in many of the foods we consume today. Fat is calorie dense at 9 calories a gram. Compared to 4 calories a gram of protein and carbohydrates, fat is the most calorie-packed macro. So 40 grams of fat would equal 360 calories. Unlike carbs, fats do not affect blood sugar levels. They do, however slow down digestion, diminishing insulin's ability to do its job. This can lead to insulin resistance, diabetes, and other metabolic disorders and diseases.

Fats are consumed through our food and then broken down into fatty acids in the blood. These fatty acids are either saturated or unsaturated. Saturated fats, often called unhealthy fats, are solid at room temperature (think butter and red meat fat), while unsaturated fats, or healthy fats, are liquid at room temperature (think olive oil and fat from fish). These fats are often stored as triglycerides, which make up most adipose (body fat) tissue. Triglycerides can increase your risk of heart disease. When fatty acids are not stored as triglycerides in body fat, they are called free fatty acids. Fat in the bloodstream is derived from either food or body fat, and most of the *energy* from fat comes from fatty acids floating around in our bloodstream. Elevated levels of *free* fatty acids put us at high risk of cardiovascular disease and can lead to insulin resistance and diabetes, high blood pressure, and obesity.

Just like protein has essential amino acids that your body cannot make, there is also a type of fat that your body cannot make and must come from food. This healthy fat is called essential fatty acids. Consuming or supplementing *essential* fatty acids has many health benefits, including helping with weight loss. We'll talk more about this in chapter 21.

Dietary fat and cholesterol are closely related. Cholesterol is important for hormone production and constructing your body's cells. Seventy-five percent of cholesterol is made by our liver, and the rest is from our diet. The liver makes all the cholesterol our bodies will ever need. If you eat too much cholesterol, especially bad cholesterol, you can damage your arteries and increase your risk of heart disease. Saturated fats and trans fats (artificial fatty acids) have a significant effect in raising blood cholesterol levels. When excess cholesterol builds up, it leads to clogged arteries.

Here's a quick explanation of the types of cholesterol:

- **LDL cholesterol (low-density lipoprotein).** Also known as the *bad* cholesterol, LDL can result in clogged arteries, heart attacks, and strokes.
- **HDL cholesterol (high-density lipoprotein).** Also known as the *good* cholesterol, HDL helps remove cholesterol from your arteries by carrying cholesterol back to your liver for disposal.

Total cholesterol. Total cholesterol is a blood test that calculates both HDL and LDL to help find out if you are at risk of heart attack, stroke, high blood pressure, diabetes, and obesity. Triglycerides are usually tested along with cholesterol; this is known as a *lipid profile*.

Fats are a great source of energy for any kind of work. They are stored as body fat for future work, and they contribute to satiety—that is, feeling full during a meal. Fats play a role in hormone production, cell formation, and other physiological body processes.

Just how much fat is needed, though, to receive these benefits? This is an important consideration because excess fat is converted to body fat and leads to obesity, disease, and disability over time. If you are already overweight or obese, then consuming fats is the last thing your body needs.

Think of it this way. Basically, there are good and bad fats, good and bad cholesterol, and free roaming fatty acids your body will use for energy or store as body fat. A bonus is that supplementing essential fatty acids may help you lose weight and maintain a long-term healthstyle. Other than essential fatty acids, it is usually detrimental to consume any kind of fat when your body has plenty of it available already. Why risk adding more fat to your body fat? Won't eating fat lessen your chances of forcing your body to use fat it has already stored for energy? Essentially, consuming fat in food is going to make your dream body more difficult to attain.

It's like this:

Do not add butter to your English muffins if there is already plenty of it stored on your buttocks!

Do not eat the English muffin unless you need energy for work!

Trimmed down to the simplest yet necessary elements, fats:

1. Provide energy for work though food and metabolizing body fat.
2. Have a caloric value of 9 calories for 1 gram.
3. Do not affect blood sugar levels in the body but can affect insulin's ability to do its job.
4. Are broken down into fatty acids, which the body uses for energy, body fat storage, and other body functions.
5. Provides insulation from the cold when stored. (This is not a benefit if you have a nice winter coat or live in a moderate climate, which nowadays is the case for most people in the world. Besides, with global warming, the last thing most humans need is a nice layer of body fat. We are not seals living in freezing water.)
6. Contain HDL cholesterol, which is good, and LDL cholesterol, which is bad. Aim to decrease your consumption of LDL-laden foods, and choose foods higher in HDL and/or add in HDL supplements.

Vitamins and Minerals

Vitamins and minerals are vital for life. They play a part in many body functions, chemical reactions, and healing that are essential for maintaining life. To make sure you are getting enough vitamins and minerals, I recommend taking a daily multivitamin and regularly eating fibrous vegetables.

Water

Water is the lifeblood of dieting. It is necessary for digestion, metabolizing nutrients, and maintaining healthy body tissues. It should be the main source of your fluid intake throughout the day.

Simply put, when it comes to nutrition, there are great and bad proteins, good and bad carbohydrates, good and bad fats, vitamins, minerals, and water. Another way you can look at it is there are high-quality and low-quality proteins based on biological value (BV). There are preferred and detrimental carbohydrates based on their glycemic rating. Fats are bad any way you look at it if you are overweight or obese, although minimal supplementation of essential fatty acids and HDL can benefit your health and weight loss goals.

Before we can go into more detail about biological value and the glycemic index, let's explore the concept of how to get fat: *fat habits*.

CHAPTER 17
How to Get Fat

Obesity is much like an infection. It starts off unnoticed, eating one too many bites of food until body fat spreads over time, eventually leading to obesity and, if untreated, to amputated body parts, disability, and early death.

To prevent a bad situation from reoccurring, we need to know what led us there in the first place. This goes for being fat, deconditioned, and lazy. I've never met a kid who dreams of being fat, living sedentary and deconditioned, or becoming lazy or indolent.

Don't get pissed . . . it's not mean to say *lazy* or *indolent*. These are the precise words to describe what leads to the state of obesity. *Lazy* by definition is "disinclined to activity or exertion: not energetic or vigorous"; "encouraging inactivity or indolence"; "moving slowly"; and "not rigorous or strict." *Indolent* "suggests a love of ease and dislike of movement or activity" (*Merriam-Webster*, 2019).

This indolent behavior is the breeding ground for obesity. The lazy or indolent person is basically running at resting metabolic rate, and any consumption of calories over that will be stored as body fat.

Nobody wants this for their future or present. To say otherwise is a lie.

So how exactly did we get so fat, anyway?

Getting started on the wrong foot is how most of us have ended up overweight. Did your parents regularly exercise, work out, and strive to eat lean and restrictively? Did the environment you grew up in support healthy living, exercise, and eating lean? It is human nature to model parents, leaders, and mentors you grow up around; you learn how to live by their example. Their habits become your habits, good or bad. Add to that the ease of living in the greatest age of technological advancement, and we've cemented our tendency toward a sedentary state, indolent behavior, reckless overeating, and unaccountable laziness that has led us to where we are now.

Blame your parents, blame the world. Just know that all the blaming, justifying, and complaining will take you to Nowhere Newland. That's a place. It's where you're at.

Getting fat starts with one extra bite of food over your daily metabolic need. It starts with engaging in 10 fewer calories of activity than your daily consumption of calories. This reoccurrence goes unnoticed at first but eventually does a full frontal in the mirror in front of you years down the road. Getting fat is a stealthy process that happens right before your eyes, and before you know it, you're obese because you're not paying enough attention to your body, you're procrastinating with exercise and restrictive eating, you've lost interest or motivation, or you never cared about it in the first place.

Becoming obese is much like the growth of a 401(k): first a dollar is deposited, then two. Soon there are hundreds of dollars and then the momentum of interest building, then compounding interest over time. Obesity starts out the same: first as a cookie, then two, then you are ten pounds heavier. As you get fatter, you become less energetic and move slower. Soon ten pounds is fifty, then a hundred. And the momentum speeds up the fattening process—as you get fatter, moving becomes difficult, and sooner or later you just cannot move or self-care. At that point, most anything you eat is excess calories leading to fat on fat, layers upon layers. It never stops until the spoon stops. A 401(k) can start out with near nothing and blossom over time as continued deposits turn into millions of dollars and a financially secure retirement. Your body will grow just the same over time if you keep depositing body fat, but the end results are inability to self-care, low quality of life, and financial ruin.

The simple truth is that we eat ourselves into a state of obesity—and some eat themselves to death. This is no joke. Ever heard of *obesity hypoventilation syndrome*, or smothering oneself in body fat? We procrastinate exercising and doing physical activity, which help ward off weight gain. We procrastinate going on a diet or doing the work necessary to burn off all that extra body fat. We refuse to deny ourselves the succulent, sweet, and tasty foods the world has to offer. We prioritize everything in life except the needs of our body. We don't put forth action toward our health and fail to give our body the attention it needs for ultimate survival and longevity. We don't spend enough, if any, of our extremely valuable time and money to prepare lean meals, work out at a gym, or invest in things that will give us a positive *return on investment* (ROI).

An ROI is investing time, money, or yourself into something and then getting back more than your initial investment. Your ROI will be a reward greater than the whole, either financially, physically, or spiritually. When it comes to your healthstyle, you'll be able to achieve a positive ROI by replacing old habits and creating new ones.

The great thing about habits is that we can eliminate, modify, or adopt habits as needed to create the life we want or desire. If you want to look like the fitness or bodybuilding person you see online or on TV, then learn and adopt their habits wholeheartedly and put them into practice indefinitely. If you want to be financially wealthy, then learn and adopt the habits of a millionaire or billionaire. If you want to be a great parent, mimic the actions and habits of a great parent you know. Many of us do not personally know or have access to successful millionaires or fitness and bodybuilding professionals, but we do have access to the books they write that lay out the habits, thinking processes, and behaviors that helped them get where they are today.

It is much easier to adopt and maintain a new habit than to eliminate a deep-seated one you want to eliminate, especially when it comes to food. Deciding to go on a weight loss program involves a twofold scenario of eliminating old detrimental habits and simultaneously learning and adopting new positive and productive habits.

It is not just a matter of habit replacement when it comes to weight loss and bodybuilding; you still have to persevere through not doing what you are comfortable doing and at the same time doing what you are uncomfortable doing—and keep doing this over and over and over again until what was comfortable becomes uncomfortable and what was uncomfortable becomes comfortable. This is the basic truth of habit changing. A habit is a ritual—like breathing, you do it without thought.

So let's take a look at some important lessons for habit forming that can help us change our obesity predicament for good. Repeat these lessons daily, weekly, and monthly to prime your body and mind for new healthy habit formation.

Lesson #1: Stop binge-watching TV shows and movies.

Imagine if you traded the time you spend binge-watching Netflix for going on walks outside, working out, or cleaning the house. How easy is it to sit down to a show and be sucked into the storyline and then sit unwavering though the whole ad-free season like it was nothing? If you trade this kind of dedication, this habit, into one that will help you lose weight and keep weight off, you will more easily live a positive healthstyle.

Lesson #2: Say no to "sweet blood."

One of the worst habits, if not the worst, that leads to obesity and ultimately severe disability or death is addiction to sugar. Sugar in the form of candy, desserts, cakes, cookies, pastries, donuts, chocolates, and the like cause hyperglycemia, or what I call *sweet blood*. This is the precursor to diabetes, artery damage, nerve damage, and a host of other negative inflictions. Sugary foods are highly addictive to our brains, and although sugar overconsumption is one of the hardest habits to kick, it's doable and necessary for you to be successful in this transformation journey.

Remember the hormone insulin we've talked about? The most powerful naturally released anabolic hormone the human body has to offer? Well, guess what? It is directly related to sweet blood. If you don't remember, anabolic is a state of growth or storing, and insulin provokes anabolism—and powerfully at that.

Insulin is released into the bloodstream by the pancreas in response to elevated blood sugar . . . sweet blood. If you took a swig of that blood, it would likely taste as sweet as syrup. The medical term for sweet blood is *hyperglycemia*: "excess of sugar in the blood" (*Merriam-Webster*). When insulin is released, the body is in storing or growing mode and helps put macronutrients (proteins, carbs, and fats) where they are needed to repair muscles and damaged body tissues, metabolize carbs and fats for energy, or store all excess calories as body fat. There are two key facts here:

1. **Insulin** is a super powerful hormone that leads to storing macronutrients quickly and promotes growth, repair, and storage. Insulin leads to *more*.

2. **Hyperglycemia/sweet blood** triggers the release of insulin, and the more the sweet, the more the insulin, and the more the insulin, the faster the conversion of macros to growth, repair, and storage. Hyperglycemia leads to insulin, which leads to *more*.

Knowing that insulin is such a powerful hormone that leads to *more*, one could say that we may need to avoid releasing insulin altogether because storing more body fat is counterproductive. Since insulin is triggered by elevated blood sugar, then elevated blood sugar needs to be prevented at all costs.

Hyperglycemia, or elevated blood sugar, is the worst state to be in during a cutting or weight loss phase of a fat-burning program. Hyperglycemia leads to insulin release, which in turn promotes growth and rapid storage of calories—and the last thing we need to be doing is trying to assimilate our calories quicker. This will lead to more body fat.

It is physiologically improbable—if not impossible—to burn body fat in a hyperglycemic state. What I mean by *improbable* is that there is a small chance that through unique physiological situations, a highly athletic and conditioned person can burn body fat in a hyperglycemic or elevated insulin state.

This happens through a complicated physiological environment of high energy consumption, high metabolism, high exertion or work, and exhaustion of all calories before they can be stored as body fat. The deconditioned fat person will have a very difficult journey attempting to tackle body fat incineration in a high blood sugar state. To avoid confusion, let's go with the idea that it is impossible to burn off body fat in a hyperglycemic state. Think of it as a ground rule to achieve the state of total body fat incineration.

This is the holy grail of fat loss right here. No shit, this is it. Remember this if you don't remember anything else: It is difficult as hell to burn off your fat ass if your blood is sweet! You can do all the cardio and weight-lifting in the world to help your muscles get stronger and grow, become better conditioned, and feel better, but you will not burn off one flipping ounce of body fat.

Workouts and cardio alone will help you look better even without any loss of body fat due to improved muscle size and tone, improved posture, and tighter skin. You will likely lower your body fat percentage, but it will not be because you burned off your body fat; it will be because you added lean muscle mass and volume through hydration and nutrient storage via glycogen (sugars stored in muscles for energy).

Lesson #3: Do not eat before bed.

Another bad habit that leads to obesity is overeating before bed, particularly carbs and fat. Overeating before bed is a great way to be fatter by morning. The body needs food for energy and recovery, but because you are doing nothing physical when you are sleeping, you don't need fat or carbohydrates in your belly at night because all those extra "energy" calories will be stored as body fat.

During sleep, you need a near empty stomach to allow your whole body to rest, including your stomach. You also need to take into account that all day you have been eating, so the food in your intestines is still being broken down and assimilated into your body.

Lesson #4: Get up early and go to bed early enough to get up early . . . every day.

Another bad habit that leads to people being overweight and obese is going to bed late and then sleeping in. Most rich, successful, in-shape, and healthy people go to bed on time and wake up earlier than everyone else, especially those involved in sports fitness, athletics, and bodybuilding. Add to this that sleeping too long is counterproductive and leaves you more fatigued with fewer awake hours of active metabolism and activity engagement.

For example, if you sleep seven hours a day, you will have seventeen hours of awake time burning calories. If you sleep ten hours, you will have fourteen active hours a day—three hours less activity eating the same number of calories. Sleeping longer automatically gives you a disadvantage over someone who sleeps less. This makes it more difficult for you to lose body fat. You can leverage this situation in your favor by going to bed early, getting six to eight hours of quality sleep, and getting up early with a ferocious, passionate readiness to engage. Rich, lean, and successful people do not sleep their lives away; they've got too much work to do and just enough time to do it.

My personal motto: "You have plenty of time to rest when you are dead."

In other words, go to bed early, get up early, and get shit done!

After waking up, exercising, writing, going to work for eight to ten hours, taking care of the kids, wife, and house, and then doing my workout, I cannot afford to sacrifice extra time to close my eyes or for that matter, watch the black hole of a boob tube.

Lesson #5: Be active and avoid sedentary time like the plague.

A habit that leads to obesity is living a sedentary lifestyle. You know by now that lack of physical activity leads to small muscles, low metabolism, and depositing excess calories as body fat. To counteract a sedentary lifestyle, you need to stop the unnecessary sedentary activities and replace them with productive activities, work, and exercise. The best way to increase your basal metabolic rate (how much fuel your body needs to stay alive) is to increase your muscle mass, but this takes time and work. You can raise your metabolism instantly by replacing your sedentary time with exercising, working out, or engaging in other exertional activities.

Repeatedly taking instant action over time increases muscle mass, the ultimate foundation to help you maintain a lean and healthy body.

Lesson #6: Avoid processed foods—aka fake foods.

People get fat because they overconsume poor-quality foods. Poor-quality foods consist of processed foods high in hydrogenated fats (unsaturated fats turned into saturated fats), high in calories, and low in protein. These foods are the ultimate fat-adding scenario. The body will not use what it does not need and will convert it into body fat. Another term I like to use for these types of food items is *fake foods* because they do not grow naturally or come from animals. They are genetically altered, machine processed, preserved to last a lifetime, and chemically enhanced to satisfy all your palatal desires. The thing that makes processed foods so bad is that they are addictive and habit forming.

Getting fat is easy. It's easy to eat too much, overconsume, choose fake foods, lie still in a recliner, and binge-watch YouTube or Netflix.

To get fat and be fat is to choose the least-resistant path in life. At least that is how it seems until you become physically disabled, diabetic, and diseased. Then your life is difficult and full of regret over inaction when you could have made a change. There comes a point when obesity is untreatable. The point of no return occurs when the comorbidities, afflictions, and medical burden overcomes the obese person, who continues to the end treading in water just trying to stay alive. Trying not to drown in their body fat, medications, pain, fatigue, and deconditioning. This usually happens when a person has been obese for a long time, becomes aged, and then loses the stamina and immunity that youth once provided. There is a consequence to every action. Indolent behavior and obesity pays a huge toll . . . a death toll.

The Ultimate Get-Fat Scenario: A Typical Example of How an Average Jane and Joe (or Marco) Get Fatter over Time

That evening, Jane and Marco sat unwavering through two episodes of *Game of Bones*, snacking on potato chips and chocolates. This was after a dinner of tacos with guacamole, sour cream, and salsa trimmed with refried beans, Spanish rice, and tapioca pudding for dessert.

With their bellies full and finally getting tired, Jane and Marco retired to the bedroom at 11:00 p.m.

Critical analysis: Tacos with trimmings and dessert will lead to obesity mainly because of the dessert, which causes hyperglycemia and consequently secretion of insulin, the growth hormone whose sole job is to store all those macronutrients. The condiments, guacamole and sour cream, are high in fat, so in the presence of insulin and the sedentary environment of watching TV, they will most likely get stored as body fat as they are not needed for work energy. If the taco meat is the typical 20 percent fat, then most of the fat calories will also be stored as body fat. The protein in the meat and beans will be used for tissue repair, muscle synthesis, and recovery and replenishment in the body. The taco shells, rice, and refried beans are carbohydrate packed, and these calories will go toward liver and muscle glycogen replenishment, organ function, and of course body fat because Jane and Marco are not physically active.

So, already this evening Jane and Marco are set up to not lose any body fat because dinner does not support weight loss, and then they really unload the obesity missiles with their post-dinner snacking. One potato chip and chocolate missile at a time, they launch the onslaught of obesity deposits and terror to their body. As the missiles of potato chips and chocolates hit the bloodstream, the radiating effects of hyperglycemia flood the environment, triggering a barrage of insulin attacks. The body has no defense against this invasion of foreign fat deposits one after another, until the landscape is doomed to be left a little thicker, puffier, and smoother by morning . . . and this was just dinner.

The next morning Jane and Marco slept in until 8:00 a.m. and then had to get ready for work.

Breakfast for Jane was a 20-ounce triple-shot white chocolate mocha with whipped cream picked up in the drive-thru on the way to work. Worse yet, Marco skips breakfast entirely.

Between clocking in to work and eating lunch, they both get hunger pangs. Marco opts for a breaktime snack, which ends up being a mocha and bagel with cheese from the coffee shop across the street. Jane eats nothing.

Critical analysis: To start, Jane and Marco overslept. Nine hours is too much sleep, especially for their sedentary lifestyles. They should have woken up at seven or eight and kick-started the day with fasted cardio, jogging, or riding a bike. They skipped a breakfast consisting of food that would have given them sustained energy for the early part of the day and kick-started their metabolisms. Instead, Jane supplemented with a high-glycemic, sugary, fat-laden drink that will lead to sweet blood, insulin surge, and an energy crash midmorning. And because Marco skipped breakfast entirely, he too has yet to kick-start his metabolism. Without morning activity or exercise, they have not jump-started their metabolisms to burn calories for the remainder of the day. Their bodies remain in the slothful state of oversleeping and inactivity from the evening before. Marco's midmorning snack to curb his hunger pangs until lunch is sugar laden, high in fat, and high in carbohydrates. Because Jane and Marco are not engaging in physically intensive manual labor jobs, their resulting hyperglycemia and insulin surges can only lead to storing extra calories as body fat and another energy crash.

At lunchtime, Jane and Marco eat lasagna, garlic bread, a small salad, and a brownie while socializing with coworkers before going back to work.

Critical analysis: Lasagna is high calorie and carbohydrate loaded with a little protein and moderate fat. This alone has enough calories and macronutrients to power Jane and Marco through the rest of their workday. But they have added in a typical side—garlic bread—which is laden with fat and carbs. This sends their moderate, lasagna-triggered insulin release into a hyperstate as white bread is similar to sugar in leading to hyperglycemia and an insulin spike.

The salad, minus any sugar-laden or fattening dressing, will balance things out a bit by decreasing the meal's *glycemic load*. But the massive surge in sweet blood that bypasses the salad's moderation and spikes the insulin levels into oblivion is all thanks to the brownie. The result of lunch is a lot of calories that will be stored rapidly due to the hyperglycemic state and insulin load. This will lead to more calories being stored as body fat and the inability for Jane and Marco to burn body fat even if they're in a calorie-restricted state. If Jane and Marco had skipped breakfast and midmorning snacks, then this would have been their first meal of the day to finally kick-start their metabolisms.

I mentioned a new term here, *glycemic load*. We know that rising blood sugar or sweet blood causes an internal reaction, which is a release of insulin in an amount corresponding to the level of hyperglycemia. The more hyperglycemia, the more insulin. The more insulin, the more rapidly proteins, carbs, and fats are assimilated. Glycemic load takes into account the meal as a whole and how it affects blood sugar and insulin response. Lasagna alone has a glycemic score of 70. When you eat a leafy green salad with lasagna, then the salad, which has a super-low glycemic score of 15, will slow the lasagna's digestion and movement through your stomach and digestive tract because it is much harder and more time consuming to digest. This will bring down the overall glycemic load of the meal. Because the salad slowed the breakdown of the lasagna, your blood sugar level will lower as will your insulin release, resulting in a lower glycemic load.

Another example is eating a couple of pieces of white bread. Bread is a high-glycemic carbohydrate with a glycemic rating of about 100, meaning it is quickly digested and assimilated into the bloodstream, leading to high blood sugar and thus a rapid and high surge of insulin. If you eat it with a beef steak, which is more difficult and time consuming to digest, this will lower the glycemic load of the meal. Steak alone has basically no blood sugar response, a glycemic rating of 0, as it has no carbohydrates, and bread alone has a rapid digestion rate and high blood sugar and insulin production, but the steak and bread combined leads to a moderate blood sugar and insulin response.

Imagine that high glycemic is water and lower glycemic is dirt. Water alone will rapidly flow through a funnel. Dirt will also fall through the funnel, just not as fast as water.

Now mix water and dirt together, which makes a thicker medium that will get through the funnel at a much slower speed. You might have to shake the funnel around to get it to go through, but at some point, the medium will flow all the way through. Now compare water to white bread and dirt to steak; the medium is the glycemic load. High-speed flow is hyperglycemia, and slow flow is minimally elevated blood sugar. The medium is thicker, denser, more complex, and harder for the funnel or digestive tract to digest.

For most people, it is not worth the time to try and calculate glycemic load. Calculating glycemic load is difficult and often inaccurate, and it is better thought of in concept. How can a formula quantify the answer as a number or score for carbohydrates of different glycemic ratings, proteins of different biological value and structure, fats of different consistency, fiber, vitamins and minerals, blood sugar, insulin, and digestion? Nope, not possible in my opinion and not necessary in the least bit for your mission to melt off all that body fat and add muscle tissue. I want you to take away the main concept of glycemic load: that if you mix complex-structured foods like meat and vegetables with simple-structured foods like breads and fruits, then the complex foods will bring down the glycemic rating of the carbs.

It is easier to concentrate on the *glycemic index* rating of each carbohydrate. The glycemic rating system for determining how a carbohydrate source affects blood sugar is pretty accurate and trustworthy. There is no way to know for sure the score for glycemic load, however. Just know that it does factor into most meals.

By the time work is through, Jane and Marco are starting to get those hunger pangs again. They head home, toss their keys on the counter, and reach into a jar of trail mix to curb their appetite until dinner. They end up consuming about cup each of trail mix consisting of peanuts, almonds, oats, raisins, chocolate chips, and coconut shavings. Jane mows the lawn and Marco finishes the laundry, dusting, and preparing dinner.

Dinner ends up being a typical American staple . . . pepperoni pizza, with a Caesar salad and homemade cookies for dessert. They grab their plates, load up, and hit the couch to vacuum in dinner and their habitual sitcom. Later they snack on candies and chocolate.

Critical analysis: The post-workday snack of one cup of trail mix is a total of about 700 calories—a calorie-dense punch to the gut. Of the 700 calories, most are from fat (peanuts, almonds, and coconut) and sugar (chocolate and raisins). There is only a negligible amount of low biological value protein from the nuts. There we go! The worst scenario of adding fat and sugar together and eating it. The consequences of this snack are a rapid spike in blood sugar, the corresponding insulin spike, and rapid storage of the fat and carbs with assimilation of the trace amount of protein. This snack results in curbing their appetites, jacking their blood sugar and insulin, and storing some of the calories as body fat because they are minimally physically active after work. This high-fat, high-sugar, high-calorie snack ignites the flame, which then sets off a nuclear barrage of a fat-laden, radiating-calorie pizza with post-sugary fallout soon to follow.

Dinner is not unusual. Pizza is super high calorie, high fat, and again high carbohydrate. There is some protein in the pepperoni but a very low amount. Pepperoni is mostly fat calories. The salad is there to say something is healthy; it's really just a condiment and will barely lower the glycemic load of the meal. The cookies on top of a bucketload of fat and carbs in the belly send the pancreas into maximal output, surging insulin to its peak. Jane and Marco are resting on the couch with about 2,000 calories apiece surging through their veins along with a boatload of insulin to help store all those calories as fast as possible. The post-dinner snacking and sedentary state is a perfect setting for storing calories as body fat. They are watching their show, happy and getting fatter. I guess this is where the saying "fat and happy" comes from.

To follow up, they go to bed later in the evening again then sleep in to the last minute possible. Sleeping at night is the most sedentary time of the day, a dead zone in the fat-burning pathway. Trust me on this one. Jane and Marco woke up fatter the next morning. This scenario happens day after day, month after month, year after year and eventually you're packing around an obese or morbidly obese body that you barely had to work for . . . or did you work hard at it? Think of all the hours a person puts into relaxing, snacking, and doing nothing day after day after day. A fat body doesn't just smack itself onto you and voila—you are obese. No. You earned it.

Getting fat is easy. We all naturally have some idea of how to get fat. Right?

Obesity is the result of:

1. Eating *too much food, too many calories,* and the *wrong foods*—fake foods, snacking, calorie-dense foods, high fat content foods, and foods low in protein.
2. Getting *too much rest.* Too much sleep adds to *sedentary behavior*—being lazy and indolent.
3. Modeling, adopting, and acting out the wrong habits. That is, practicing *get-fat habits vs. get-lean-and-stay-lean habits.* Modeling obese or overweight parents, obese teachers, and poor-quality mentors. Or perhaps you had good role models, but the lack of results prove you didn't gain the necessary knowledge on health and wellness during your developmental years.

Uncontrolled blood sugar, excessive insulin, and reckless consumption of fats and sugars. In other words, maintaining a physiological state that prevents fat burning and promotes body fat storage.

This means that even if you are exercising or working out after a meal, depending on the meal and the effects it has on your blood sugar and insulin levels, you can still get fatter.

So, we're frickin' doomed, right?

Guess what! There is a solution to prevent this scenario and get the opposite effect.

You can create an environment within your body to burn off fat and lose weight—and you don't even have to exercise. No shit.

I call it *the State*.

The State (*status burnfaticus*): "Creating an environment in your body that prevents storage of body fat and in turn leads to metabolizing calories for energy, synthesizing calories for repair and replenishment, and ultimately pulling from body fat storage in an energy deficit."

Simply put, if you eat this and do that, *in the State*, you force your body to suck all the fat out of your fat ass, beer belly, thunder thighs, and double chin and incinerate then excrete it. Do this over and over again, day after day, week after week, month after month, and depending on your level of obesity, sooner or later all your excess body fat will be gone . . . all of it.

So how does a person achieve this? How do you get into a state of fat burning?

CHAPTER 18
Low-Glycemic Carbohydrates

EATING CARBOHYDRATES CAUSES a rise in blood sugar leading to hyperglycemia—sweet blood—which then triggers an insulin response. How high an insulin response is corresponds to how much glucose is in the blood, and how much glucose is in the blood can be estimated by the glycemic rating of the carbohydrate. The glycemic rating of a carbohydrate rates how a carbohydrate will affect your blood sugar level and corresponding insulin response. To understand how we can use this knowledge to our advantage, to achieve the State, we need to first understand the glycemic index and how it works.

The glycemic index is a table that lists the glycemic rating for each different carbohydrate source. This score is based on how the carbohydrate affects blood sugar. The higher the rating, the higher the effect on blood sugar and the aftereffects thereof. The lower the rating, the less the effect on blood sugar and the lower the insulin response.

The glycemic index (GI) was invented in the early 1980s by David Jenkins, PhD as a tool for diabetics to help control their blood sugar. Diabetics have a predisposition to hypo- (low) or hyper- (high) glycemia, low or high blood sugar. The GI rates carbohydrates as low as 0 and as high as 100.

A low-glycemic carbohydrate will enter the bloodstream at a slow rate, preventing hyperglycemia, and stimulating only a small amount of insulin, thus preventing rapid storage of calories. A high-glycemic carbohydrate is broken down and digested quickly, leading to a state of hyperglycemia, therefore triggering a high amount of insulin in the blood and a rapid assimilation of calories.

When it comes to carbohydrates, insulin's primary job in the body is to grab up glucose molecules in the bloodstream and store them as muscle glycogen (energy stored in muscles), liver glycogen (energy stored in the liver), or body fat. Chronic high levels of insulin in the blood also triggers an onslaught of many diseases, including type 1 and type 2 diabetes, heart disease, and possibly cancer. A high-glycemic meal is also responsible for feelings of hunger due to the rapid spike and then drop in blood sugar levels, thus signaling the body to eat so it can raise blood sugar levels back to normal. The human body is constantly working to return all its chemicals to baseline or resting levels.

Carbohydrates are rated from low to high depending on how fast they are assimilated and converted into glucose in the bloodstream. Simple sugars like honey, syrups, juices, and fruits; sugary flour products like cookies and cakes; puffed rice and other processed cereals; and other similar carbs enter and then pass through the stomach quickly, leading to rapid assimilation and high blood sugar levels. These fast carbs have a high glycemic rating. Low-glycemic carbs like beans, yams, oatmeal, bran, brown rice, sweet potatoes, fructose from fruits, broccoli, lettuce, asparagus, cauliflower, celery, corn, carrots, peas, and other similar carbs sit in the stomach longer, take longer to break down, and have a slow, almost timed, release of glucose into the bloodstream. This slower, timed release results in lower blood sugar levels, which in turn leads to lower insulin response. Another way to think of consuming low-glycemic carbohydrates is as a preventive measure against high blood sugar.

It makes total sense to avoid high-glycemic carbohydrates at all costs to prevent weight gain, obesity, and the negative consequences of high blood sugar and insulin with it. Since low-glycemic carbs provide sustained energy and have less of a chance to be stored as body fat, then low-glycemic carbs are the best of all carbohydrates, period.

Now it boils down to figuring out what carbs are high, moderate, or low glycemic and when to consume carbs to get lean. To determine what the glycemic rating of a carbohydrate is, there are many sources, tables, and charts available in books and online that include a list of some of the most common carbohydrates and their subsequent glycemic ratings to get you started.

If you want more information on the glycemic index, then I recommend the *NIH News in Health* post "Counting Carbs?: Understanding Glycemic Index and Glycemic Load" from December 2012, which you can find online. A great free resource for the glycemic index can be found in the American Diabetes Association (ADA) *Diabetes Care* article "International Tables of Glycemic Index and Glycemic load Values: 2008"; see the first supplemental table. If this list is too huge, then under the Figures & Tables tab is a condensed glycemic index table and link to a PDF to download. Also see the tabs Article, Supplemental Material, and Info & Metrics, which have resources for you to use. As far as when to consume carbs, we'll get to that in chapter 20.

Aside from these online tools, I highly recommend purchasing a book that lists the details of all foods, including calories, protein, carbs, fats, sugars, sodium, potassium, the glycemic rating, and the biological value (BV) of proteins. Having this reference when you need it will be a valuable tool in your healthstyle development. This information will help you figure out meal structure and planning as well, which is necessary in your weight loss and physique transformation journey. You can use the glycemic index to make sure the carbs you are eating are indeed low glycemic, which will help you in your weight loss journey. I've provided a GI chart at the end of this chapter.

Let's look at our fictitious couple, Jane and Marco, to find out how a meal's glycemic ratings can make or break your journey toward body transformation.

Jane and Marco sat down for dinner, cracked open soda pops, and went to it while watching their favorite TV sitcom. Dinner consisted of spaghetti and meatballs, garlic butter breadsticks, Caesar salad, and brownies for dessert. Again, a typical meal.

Critical analysis: To kick things off, drinking any sugary drink including fruit juice, punch, and soda pop starts digestion as soon as the liquid touches your tongue and oral cavity.

GLYCEMIC INDEX

High Glycemic

The "Ose's"	Cornflakes: 119	French Fries: 107
Maltose: 150	Instant Potatoes: 118	Graham Wafers: 106
Glucose: 137	Rice Krispies:	Corn Chips: 105
Sucrose: 92	Pretzels: 116	Puffed Wheat: 105
Fructose: 32	Jelly Beans: 114	Mashed Potato: 104
Lactose: 15-30	Wheat bread: 112	Kaiser Rolls: 104
	Rice Cakes: 110	Watermelon: 103
Maltodextrin: 137	Vanilla Wafers: 110	White Bagel: 103
Instant Rice: 128	Waffles: 109	Carrots: 101
Baked Potato: 121	Doughnut: 108	White Bread: 100

Medium Glycemic

Mashed Potato: 100	Durum Spaghetti: 78
Cream of Wheat: 100	Sweet Corn: 78
Shredded Wheat: 99	Buckwheat: 78
Wheat Bread: 99	Oat Bran: 78
Cornmeal: 98	Sweet Potato: 77
High Fiber Wheat Bread: 97	Banana: 77
Taco Shells: 97	Quick-Cook Wheat: 77
Croissant: 96	Bulger Bread: 75
Gnocchi: 95	Canned Lentils: 74
Angel Food Cake: 95	Canned Kidney Beans: 74
Semolina: 94	Orange Juice: 74
Canned Green Pea Soup: 94	Yams: 73
Pineapple: 94	Cracked Barley: 72
Steamed Potato: 93	Cheese Tortellini: 71
Cantaloupe: 93	Lowfat Ice Cream: 71
Couscous: 93	Pumpernickel: 71
Black Bean Soup: 92	Chocolate: 70
Macaroni and Cheese: 92	Skittles: 70
Rye Bread: 92	Canned Baked Beans: 69
Beets: 91	Grapefruit Juice: 69
Raisons: 91	Mixed Grain Bread: 69
Muffins: 88	Green Peas: 68
Canned Potato: 87	Bulgur: 68
Ice Cream: 87	Instant Noodles: 67
Oatmeal: 87	Cornflakes: 81
Hamburger Bun: 87	Boiled White Potato: 80
Rice Milk: 86	Mango: 80
Split Pea Soup: 86	Popcorn: 79
Cheese Pizza: 86	Fruit Cocktail: 79
Rice Vermicelli: 86	Oatmeal Cookies: 79
Honey: 83	Instant Oatmeal: 79
White Pita Bread: 82	Brown Rice: 79

GLYCEMIC INDEX
Medium... Continued

Canned Peaches: 67
Pineapple Juice: 66
Grapes: 66
Instant Rice: 65-
Popcorn: 65
Linguine: 65
Capellini: 64
Canned Pinto Beans: 64
Sweet Potato: 63
Canned Lentil Soup: 63
Canned Pears: 63
Orange: 63
Canned Chick Peas: 60
Fresh Peach: 60
White Spaghetti: 59
Black-Eyed Beans: 59
Soda Pop/Soft Drinks: 59
Canned Chick Peas: 58
Apple Juice: 58
Durum Meat-Filled Ravioli: 56
Pinto Beans: 55
Plum: 55

Barley Kernel Bread: 55
Udon Noodles: 55
Rolled Oats/Oatmeal: 55
Brown Beans: 54
Apple: 54
Whole Grain Spaghetti: 53
Fresh Pear: 53
Specialty Grain Bread: 53
Spaghetti: 52
Chapatti: 52
Candy Bars: 51
Ice Cream: 51
Taffy: 51
Yogurt: 51
Whole Grain Spaghetti: 53
Fresh Pear: 53
Specialty Grain Bread: 53
Spaghetti: 52
Chapatti: 52
Candy Bars: 51
Ice Cream: 51
Taffy: 51
Yogurt: 51

Low Glycemic

Vermicelli: 50
Vegetable Soup: 48
Rye: 48
Chick Peas: 47
Garbanzo Beans: 47
Lowfat Low Sugar Yogurt: 47
Corn Tortilla: 46
Fettucine: 46
Frozen Baby Lima Beans: 46
Skim Milk: 46
Boiled Yellow Split Peas: 45
Butter Beans: 44
Apricots: 44
Black Beans: 43
Dates: 42
Green Lentils: 42
Kidney Beans: 42
Coconut Milk: 41
Lentils: 41
Dried Beans: 40

Regular Milk: 40
Boiled Carrots: 39
Red Lentils: 36
Grapefruit: 36
Pearled Barley: 36
Brown Beans: 34
Soy Milk: 34
Dried Peas: 32
Cherries: 32
Red Kidney Beans: 27
Rice Bran: 27
Almond Milk: 25
Soya Beans: 25
Peanuts: 21

Other Products:

Sugar Free Popsicles: 15
Sugar Free Cotton Candy: 2
Diet Soda/Diet Soft Drinks: 0

Simple sugars begin digesting in saliva, triggering the release of more saliva, stomach acids, and gastrointestinal motility. Liquid-form simple sugars like the soda pop Jane and Marco sipped on during dinner have a high glycemic rating of at least 70 because the soda passes through the stomach and GI system rapidly, turning into glucose in the bloodstream and resulting in elevated blood sugars. Already it's a doomed meal because it is physiologically unlikely to burn body fat with sweet blood, let alone that the rapid release of insulin that follows will trigger growth and rapid storage of macronutrients, including any excess calories as body fat.

Spaghetti is made of flour, sometimes eggs, and water and in its final processed form has a low to moderate glycemic rating of 50-plus. Spaghetti is broken down and assimilated into the bloodstream as glucose. Spaghetti sauce is usually low calorie and has a negligible effect on blood sugar, although many brands add a significant amount of sugar. Meatballs are mostly protein and fat, so they will have a negligible effect on blood sugar levels and will be broken down into amino and fatty acids in the bloodstream. Caesar salad dressing is high fat and high sugar and so is quickly digested and assimilated into the bloodstream as fatty acids and glucose. The vegetables in the salad are low calorie and have near zero effect on blood sugar. The brownies kick the already high blood sugar and insulin levels into overdrive. Brownies are also calorie dense and really kick the overall calories of the meal into excess. Although the green leafy vegetables from the salad and the protein from the meatballs help lower the glycemic load of the meal, this is insignificant as the overall calories of the meal are from high-glycemic carbohydrates and fat. The soda, pasta, salad dressing, and brownies are unnecessary energy during the couple's sedentary TV watching. The overall scenario of their high-carbohydrate, high-blood sugar, insulin-promoting meal leaves the couple with zero chance at losing weight. Most of the calories from this dinner will be stored as additional body fat.

Now let's look at the results of a meal with low-glycemic carbohydrates.

Jane and Marco sat down for dinner, cracked open their diet sodas, and went to it while watching their favorite TV sitcom. Dinner consisted of lean peppercorn beefsteak, grilled sweet potato wedges, asparagus, and apples for dessert.

Critical analysis: Diet sodas have zero calories. Artificial sweeteners can be considered to have a high glycemic rating, but with zero calories and in such small portions, they have a negligible and short-lived blood sugar response. When compared to regular soda, diet soda is like water and regular soda is liquid sugar. Diet soda is a much healthier alternative to any sort of sugar water. Beefsteak is a protein-dense food with zero carbs and does not affect blood sugar directly. (Indirectly, beefsteak without carbs will trigger the liver to release stored sugars into the bloodstream and a corresponding insulin response, promoting digestion and assimilation of the protein and fat. The liver will release only the amount of glucose necessary for the protein.) Peppercorns have a null effect on blood sugar.

Sweet potatoes have a low glycemic rating of 46 if boiled, and grilling will likely raise the GI negligibly. Due to their low glycemic rating, they will have a low insulin result when broken down into glucose, leading to a more timed released or delayed assimilation and storage of calories. This means more of the glucose will be used as energy storage as muscle glycogen and liver glycogen and as energy for metabolism. Asparagus is a low-glycemic fibrous carbohydrate with a rating of 8. The asparagus in this meal will even further delay digestion due to the fibrous makeup, low calories, and trace effect on blood sugar. Again, another food promoting a timed-release effect of the whole meal.

The apple is low glycemic with a rating of 39, at about 95 calories. The apple results in a low glycemic response and thus low insulin levels. Its simple sugars will be converted to glucose rapidly, but the fibrous parts will also aid in slowing the meal's digestion and assimilation.

Here's another way to look at low-glycemic carbs compared to high-glycemic carbs: Imagine eating a 2,000-calorie meal in one sitting. A high-glycemic, 2,000-calorie meal will have a ton of insulin and fast assimilation of, let's say, two hours, whereas a low-glycemic, 2,000-calorie meal will have a low-insulin environment and a slow assimilation of, let's say, six hours. Two thousand calories assimilated into the body in two hours at 1,000 calories per hour (CPH) will lead to more excess of calories over the body's metabolic rate, so they will be converted to and stored as body fat.

Two thousand calories assimilated into the body over six hours—three times faster—will at a rate of 333 CPH (1,000 divided by three) have a much lower chance of exceeding the body's caloric needs and therefore a much lower chance of storing calories as body fat. Let's look at this math a little closer.

How to Figure Your Calories per Hour Speed Limit

Just like all roads and highways have a speed limit, your body has a calorie limit based on metabolism. How active you are and what type of work you do while you're awake determines your metabolic or caloric need. If you are doing nothing all day, then your calorie limit will be low because your body does not need that much energy or fuel to function. If you are active, exercise, engage in manual labor, and avoid sedentary time, then your calorie limit will be much higher because your body needs fuel for work.

Since consuming low-glycemic versus high-glycemic carbohydrates will directly affect the time it takes to digest, assimilate, and use or store the calories, it is vital to make sure you are staying within your speed limit, or your metabolic calorie limit per hour.

To prevent getting fatter.

What is your body's speed limit?

How many calories an hour can you go before you get a big fat speeding ticket?

First, you need to figure out how many awake hours of the day you have (twenty-four hours – sleep time = awake time), then divide your basal metabolic rate by awake hours (BMR/awake hours = calories per hour limit). This is your CPH at a minimum based on BMR. If you add in all the extra calories needed for exercise like weightlifting and other extracurricular activities, then your CPH will be higher than if you're operating at BMR.

You can use the *Harris-Benedict equation* to determine your total daily caloric need or otherwise stated, your basal metabolic rate.

Harris-Benedict Equation to calculate basal metabolic rate (BMR)

Women: BMR = 655 + (4.35 x Weight in lbs.) + (4.7 x Height in inches) - (4.7 x Age in Years)

Men: BMR = 66 + (6.2 x Weight in lbs.) + (12.7 x Height in inches) - (6.76 x Age in Years)

Now that you know your BMR, you can figure out your calorie per hour limit based on awake hours.

Your BMR is your metabolism setup point without added work or exercise. You can figure out how many calories will exceed your BMR by adding the calories you estimate you'll be burning to your BMR. This is referred to as your total daily calorie (or energy) expenditure. For example, you would add 700 calories for one hour on the elliptical or 250 calories for walking an hour.

The formula for this is:

BMR + extra calories burned form work/exercise

= total daily energy expenditure (TDEE)

Now figure out your speed limit, your calories per hour (CPH), by dividing your TDEE by your awake hours:

TDEE/awake hours = calories per hour (CPH)

If you cannot estimate how many extra calories you need to add for work or exercise, the Mifflin-St. Jeor formula can help you calculate your TDEE:

BMR × activity level = TDEE

Mifflin St. Jeor Equation: (TDEE)

Women: BMR = (10 x Weight in kg) + (6.25 x height in cm) - (5 x Age in years) - 161

Men: BMR = (10 x Weight in kg) + (6.25 x Height in cm) - (5 x Age in years) +5

The most important number to look at here is your BMR. If your goal is to burn body fat, then how many extra calories you burn from work or exercise is irrelevant. If you calculate the exercise and work into your total daily energy expenditure needs, you will likely end up overestimating and consuming too many calories—which obviously prevents weight loss. It is more important to focus on your BMR, then consider any extra work or exercise a bonus because a calorie deficit from your TDEE is what makes the body pull from its fat stores for energy.

Remember, this is the ultimate goal: to make your body eat its own fat using internal mechanisms of the metabolic process. We know the body will not eat its own body fat in a high blood sugar state, so it is vital to keep our blood sugar as low as possible. We can accomplish this by choosing low-glycemic carbohydrates or no carbohydrates at all.

So, now we understand the benefit of low-glycemic carbs versus high-glycemic carbs and the benefits of using the glycemic index in meal planning. We also learned about the body's speed or calorie limit per hour and how to calculate it based on industry standard formulas. Now it's time to move further with our healthstyle transformation using *high biological value*, or BV protein rating. What is it, and how can you use it to improve your chances at getting lean and healthy?

CHAPTER 19
High Biological Value (BV) Proteins

When it comes to choosing what protein sources to eat, the BV rating, or biological value score, of a protein source can help you decide. Every protein has a score that corresponds to how well that protein source is assimilated into the body for repair, replenishment, and muscle synthesis. A protein with low biological value will have less value for your body as far as being assimilated for structural repair, hormonal replenishment, or building new tissues. Conversely, a protein with high biological value has a better chance at being assimilated for growth, repair, and replenishment. For example, a whole raw soybean has a low BV because it is difficult for the body to digest due to the tough husk shell coating and structural makeup—in fact, it is actually a carbohydrate product, unlike soy isolate protein powder. Soy protein isolate is a source of protein and is high BV because it is easily assimilated and used for protein's many jobs in the body.

Nitrogen is a basic component of amino acids. As we mentioned in a previous chapter, amino acids are put together by the body to make up all the necessary protein structures. Since nitrogen makes up the bulk of amino acids, it's a significant factor to measure in BV.

How can nitrogen be measured? *Nitrogen in versus nitrogen out* reveals how much nitrogen remains in, and how much nitrogen remains in determines how usable the protein source is for the body. Nitrogen out is how unusable the protein is for the body. This is what the biological value (BV) score refers to—how valuable a protein source is in the human body and the predictable chance that it will be used and not converted to waste.

Whether a person is in a state of maintenance, growth, or tissue healing, the replenishment from protein assimilation and use is referred to as being in a *positive nitrogen state*. If a person is in a *negative nitrogen state*, they are likely protein deficient and in a decaying, catabolic/cannibolic, fasting/starving, and/or sarcopenic (wasting of skeletal muscle mass) state. Given this, typical human beings, from birth to death, should do everything within their power to stay in a positive nitrogen state, especially when on a weight loss plan or fasting.

To burn off body fat, we must consume fewer calories than we metabolize. In other words, we need to have a negative calorie deficit. Fasting at its core is consuming water and zero calories from food. It is the ultimate state of being in a negative calorie deficit—in fact, 100 percent of your energy and protein needs will be taken from your body when you fast. It's purely catabolic or cannibalism, in a way, eating or metabolizing yourself from the inside out, consuming your own body tissues to maintain life. But 100 percent fasting for too long leads to starvation, and this is a road to mortality as your body eats itself to death. Obviously, that is not recommended. You want to avoid both metabolizing and starving yourself to death.

The last thing we want while on a diet is to cannibalize or metabolize our lean muscle tissue because this leads to a lower resting metabolic rate, loss of strength, and decreased immunity. So when you're on a diet with the goal to lose body fat, you need to do a little fasting to put yourself in a calorie deficit while preserving lean muscle tissue.

I've said it before—you cannot lose all your body fat by exercise alone. This perpetuating myth needs to be dispelled. You can do all the aerobics, calisthenics, sports, or weightlifting you want, but you will never get lean if your nutritional environment does not support fat burning. Remember, it is physiologically impossible to burn body fat in a hyperglycemic state because of the presence of insulin. Many research studies conclude that elevated insulin (the most powerful growth hormone) prevents the burning of body fat. Since sugar in the blood in any amount leads to an insulin response, it is clear that we must prevent insulin release to achieve a state of fat burning. It is logical to say, then, that we will not burn fat in a hyperglycemic, high blood sugar, or sweet blood state. Other factors prevent fat burning, too, including being in a calorie surplus and timing of macronutrient consumption, including protein consumption.

To make sure we are in a positive nitrogen state at all times, especially when on a weight loss or fasting program, we need to consume an adequate amount of protein, and that protein needs to be valuable. This is where the BV scale comes into play. We can use it to choose high BV proteins for the bulk of our meals and daily consumption. Because high-BV protein consumption accelerates and promotes a positive nitrogen state during fasting and calorie restriction, exercise is an added bonus to burn off even more body fat, turning your body into a fat-ass incinerator. The *EXER* in EXERLEAN.

Let's look at an example of nitrogen with Jane and Marco, who have decided to go on a diet to lose weight.

Jane is now a vegetarian. Using the Harris-Benedict formula, she has learned that her BMR is about 1,600 calories a day. Being a vegetarian, she will be getting the bulk of her protein from carbohydrate sources like beans, nuts, wheat, and rice. She plans to consume four 300-calorie meals a day for a total of 1,200 calories. This puts her in a calorie deficit of 400 calories a day. This seems like a good plan that should lead to a 2,800-calorie deficit a week, almost a one-pound-a-week deficit (3,500 fewer calories equals about a pound of weight lost). In addition, any extra exercise or activity will contribute to a higher negative calorie deficit, leading to even more weight loss. If Jane runs forty-five minutes every day on the treadmill, this will add -500 calories (-3,500 a week) to her daily weight loss, which turns the 2,800-calorie deficit from dieting alone to a 6,300-calorie deficit. That's now over a two-pound-a-week weight loss scenario.

Critical analysis: The problem in this situation is the protein from Jane's carbohydrate sources is low biological value and an insufficient amount. Carbohydrate sources of protein like soy, other beans, and grains are exactly that—mostly carb calories. There is very little protein in these carbohydrate foods; therefore, they are a poor-quality protein source of low biological value. In this scenario, Jane is going to be in a negative nitrogen balance because of lack of protein, period. Being in a negative nitrogen balance, Jane will burn much of her muscle tissue right along with body fat. She is in more of a wasting state, and after a month of this program, she will have lost about two pounds a week for a total of eight pounds in the month, but of the eight pounds lost, much will be muscle tissue . . . pounds of it gone. A month later, with pounds of muscle tissue obliterated, her BMR is now lower, making it even harder to burn off body fat. She also has less muscle bulk for work, has less energy, and likely feels like shit. If she keeps up this scenario, she will likely get sick and end up in the hospital for malnutrition, sarcopenia, or some other wasting disease.

Let's fix Jane's situation by using high BV protein. Going on a diet, Jane is now in a fasting state or negative calorie deficit, and her body needs extra protein to remain in a positive nitrogen state. The fact is that being on a vegetarian diet does make it difficult to achieve an anabolic or positive nitrogen state in a calorie-restricted, high-carbohydrate environment because vegetarians basically eliminate all the high BV proteins in their diets except soy protein isolate. Soy protein isolate, derived from soybeans, is pure protein minus the carbs and has a high biological value.

Jane has a BMR of 1,600 calories. She has opted to do a four-meal split a day at 300 calories a meal for a total of 1,200 calories a day, creating a 400-calorie deficit from diet and another 500 calories a day from exercise. She opts to consume soy protein isolate as half of those calories. Now Jane has half of her calories coming from high BV protein. This scenario leads to higher nitrogen levels and a better chance to preserve her lean muscle tissue, with an end result of losing eight pounds, more of which is body fat and not muscle mass. Now, on to Marco.

Marco uses the Harris-Benedict formula and calculates a BMR of 2,400 calories. Marco decides to use a four-meal split of 500 calories a meal for a total of 2,000 calories a day. He also plans to exercise daily, forty-five minutes on the treadmill, for a total of -500 calories a day. Calorie restriction and exercise combined leads to a 900-calorie-a-day deficit for a 6,300-calorie-a-week deficit, which should result in nearly two pounds a week of weight loss. He plans to consume a high-protein diet using high-BV protein sources including egg whites, beef, chicken, and casein-and-whey-protein shakes. Marco is going to be consuming high BV protein in every meal from wake to sleep. In this scenario, Marco will be in a positive nitrogen state throughout most of the day and will have the benefits of anabolism with it.

In Jane's and Marco's two high BV scenarios, there are many other variables that come into play, such as when you start adding fasting, carb depletion, protein loading, and fasted exercise, but these are good examples of the difference between being in a positive nitrogen and negative nitrogen state because of type and quantity of protein intake.

Pulling It All Together

It is now time to summarize the lessons we have learned and seat them into our memory banks.

We started out in the beginning of this book with a slap in the face, the human cattle prod I call it, focusing on the negative effects of obesity and how obesity is making your life hell, which will only get worse with age. I opened your eyes to the current state of the obesity epidemic. With so much negativity around the state of obesity, every person needs to take a stance against it, get rid of it, and prevent it at all costs to enhance and preserve life. We talked about the laws and principles of Bodinomics: the economy of the human body, and how you can use the cost-benefit analysis to make the right decisions in life, especially when dealing with what to eat, what not to eat, work performance, and exercise. Your activities of daily living, behaviors, habits, and actions determine your healthstyle and quality-of-life status.

We learned about the benefits of exercise and fasted exercise and how timing of calorie intake and exercise can lead to different fat-burning outcomes. We have talked about the benefits of weight training, strengthening, and my custom workout format, Weight Chaining. Chaining is a two-day workout split separating the body's anterior and posterior chains and achieves a full-body workout in just two days, which also promotes extension of the body against gravity. We talked about EXERPAIN and how to deal with it, then persevere through your transformation journey. We went through different scenarios on how to get fat to better understand how we can become obese so easily, which will help us change our behaviors and habits and prevent them from entering our healthstyles. We have discussed the negative results of hyperglycemia, or sweet blood, and how it will prevent fat burning and lead to other negative body diseases, then decay. We also learned how to use the glycemic index to choose low-glycemic carbs to help us prevent hyperglycemia and maintain low blood sugar, leading to better metabolic outcomes. Finally, we learned the importance of maintaining a positive nitrogen state to achieve health and wellness and especially when in a state of fasting, intermittent fasting, or dieting to prevent muscle wasting.

Now, let's get into how you can strategically use low-glycemic carbs, high biological value proteins, weight training, and fasted exercise to achieve a state of ultimate fat-burning and physique transformation and get in the best shape of your life—and remain there indefinitely.

We have come to the source, the secret body-fat-burning algorithm, the State. How to achieve and master the state of thermogenesis. This is body fat incineration at its maximum velocity.

**It's time to become master and controller over your body.
"Let's do this!"**

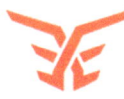 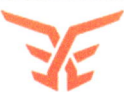

"The BV Scale"
Bioavailability of Protiens

Whey Protein Isolate: 100-159
Whey Protein Concentrate: 104
Whole Egg: 100
Whey Protein: 96
Whole Bean: 96
Whole Soy Bean: 96
Breast Milk (human): 95
Cow Milk: 91
Soy Milk: 91
Egg Whites: 88
Cheese: 84
Quinoa: 83
Chicken/Turkey: 79
Casein-: 77
Fish: 76-83
Lean Beef: 74-80

Soy Protein Powder: 74
Soy Beans: 73
Oats: 66
Rice: 64-83
Soy Flour: 64-81
Tofu: 64
Whole Wheat/Grains/Gluten: 64
Wheat: 54
Beans: 49
Soy Beans: 47
Peanuts: 43-55
White Flour: 41
Corn: 36
Dry Beans: 34
White Potato: 34

BV = Retained/Absorbed
BV = (Intake-Fecal-Urine)/Intake-Fecal
Nitrogen in VS Nitrogen out-

CHAPTER 20
The State

THERE ARE MANY ways to skin a rattlesnake, and the same goes with the path to weight loss. Skilled wrestlers can lose over ten pounds in one day to make their weight class by depleting sodium and glycogen stores and sweating away water volume. This is an extreme example of weight loss and not your goal, yet it shows that there are many ways to lose body weight. You have a multitude of weight loss plans at your discretion, some with polarizing ideas about cutting calories, cutting carbs, cutting fat, or cutting sugar; others that are gluten-free, meat-free, fruit-free, or food-free; and many with whatever plethora of other methods are at your disposal.

The truth is simple—eating fewer calories than your basal metabolic rate (BMR) will lead to weight loss. Cutting carbs is one of the quickest methods. Switching to a low-fat diet may lead to weight loss over time, but you must be in a calorie deficit. You may lose weight on a juice, grapefruit, ketogenic, low-carb, vegetarian, tuna, gluten-free, TV-icon, fad, or tabloid diet, from prepackaged meal-plan programs, and a billion other options but all with varying levels of positive and possibly negative outcomes.

Some weight loss programs work much better than others at helping you burn off body fat. Some weight loss plans will actually make you fatter. Some focus on weight loss at all costs regardless of where the weight is being taken from, even if it's from lean body mass or muscle tissue. Remember, loss of lean body mass or burning off muscle tissue in a fasting state is the worst possible outcome of your weight loss journey.

I've experimented with many different programs, methods, diet plans, and unique ideas to lose weight. A common theme I have noticed is that the diet and weight loss programs that feel less restricted focus more on personal enjoyment than on results and lead to poor outcomes. And vice versa—the most restrictive and less comfortable pathways tend to lead to the best fat-burning results. This is subjective, though, because what one person feels is restrictive might feel comfortable to another, and what feels comfortable or enjoyable to one might feel gluttonous to another.

When a person has been on a restrictive diet long enough to make it habitual, then cheating, overeating, or consuming off-diet foods does not feel or even taste good. This is because they have forgotten about all the bad eating habits and hyperpalatable food addictions. If you eat restrictively and lean long enough to make it the new baseline, then when you do eat processed, high-fat, or sugary foods, they will taste abnormal and make you feel like crap. Eating restrictively also leads to a healthier body and a better sense of well-being. When you develop a positive and restrictive healthstyle, you increase self-control, confidence, and pride. When you take care of your body, engage in positive activities, and eat for longevity, health, and wellness, then only good can result. Your routine diet is likely the most powerful platform from which all other aspects of physical and mental wellness develop in your life.

Some people can't stand the word *diet* for many reasons, but it is the perfect word to use when describing how and what you eat on a regular basis. The word *diet* is not limited to a weight loss program, plan, or eating protocol. It pertains to all human beings. We each have our own personal food choices and feeding routine, and this is referred to as our diet. According to the dictionary, a diet is "food and drink regularly provided or consumed"; "habitual nourishment: the kind and amount of food prescribed for a person or animal for a special reason"; "a regimen of eating and drinking sparingly so as to reduce one's weight"; "something provided or experienced repeatedly" (*Merriam-Webster*).

Some of us have chosen to share our own diets with the world in books, videos, pictures, and programs. I have spent decades putting together this book to share my personal diet with you because plain and simple, it gets the job done!

EXERLEAN takes what works and incorporates it into the program. Anything else, the stuff that doesn't work or has lackluster results, has been eliminated to save you time. EXERLEAN combines the best methods of fat burning with the best formulas for lean mass preservation and strengthening, with the overarching goal to help you design, adopt, and maintain maximal health status. EXERLEAN incorporates secret dieting protocols that competitive bodybuilders use to achieve atypical extraordinary results.

Your time is valuable and nonrefundable. We must make every minute count toward positive, productive, and rewarding outcomes.

You need to understand that no one specific method or diet will work for the long term. The best long-term results come from a program that involves using different methods of varying, cycling, fasting, and refeeding. This is because the body will adapt to any specific method after a certain engagement time. This time of adaption is usually when results start to diminish. Not that diminishing results is a bad thing because the same method used indefinitely will eventually lead to a state of maintenance. At that point, if you are in great shape, strong, energetic, and happy, then maintenance is a good thing. Maintenance is not the preferred scenario if you are still overweight and dealing with folds of fat waiting to be burned, or if you have potential to get stronger, lack vitality, lack happiness, and continue to desire change. Progression, not maintenance, is then your goal. Variation prevents adaption and promotes continued changes in your body, which can help prevent you from plateauing or bust you out of a plateau. EXERLEAN: the State is designed to keep your body guessing and changing for the better, to prevent plateaus, and to help you maintain the results of your hard work for the long term.

The State is when your body is forced to burn pure body fat for energy at a maximal rate. When the State has been achieved, the body is forced to devour its own body fat through the metabolic pathway. Achieving the State of ultimate body fat incineration takes a disciplined and focused approach. All the steps and criteria must be met for a successful outcome. It is complicated science, but I've simplified it in this book. Coming up is the detailed plan on how to get yourself into the State, remain there as long as beneficial, and get out when necessary. All you have to do is follow the plan and do not derail, cheat, or sabotage your mission.

The State of ultimate body fat incineration is an EXERLEAN algorithm that's two weeks long and easy to follow. Remember, the best things in life are not easy to garner but are forged in time by your inner blacksmith.

Ultimately, you make you. Your body is the result of your exercising and eating choices over the course of time. The environment you live in, your daily routine, and the people who surround you was and is created by you.

Envision your future self and do the work necessary to make future you a reality. This is just a guide to help you get there faster.

The three-step process to achieve the perfect state of fat burning.

To turn you into a body fat incinerator . . .

EXERLEAN Fat-Burning Algorithm

Step One: Glycogen Depletion

Days 1 through 2, 3, or 4

Goal: Deplete muscle and liver glycogen. Achieve a baseline nutritional state, or *clean the slate*. We need to empty the tank before we can fill it with only the specific macronutrient profile that turns the body into a fat-burning furnace.

Carb depletion is the process used to achieve glycogen depletion. Carb depletion means that we stop consuming 100 percent carbohydrates, including sugars, fruits, grains, and vegetables. To accomplish this is simple—just stop eating carbs and anything containing carbs, period. That leaves you with protein or fat to eat. Eating fat is bad but not so much so in the case of carb depletion. The goal of carb depletion is to achieve a state of muscle and liver glycogen depletion, taking the body to the brink of ketosis.

So, what is ketosis?

Ketosis is when all muscle and liver glycogen has been used up for energy, then the body starts to convert body fat into ketone bodies, which are then used as energy for work, activity, or exercise. The point at which ketone bodies are released into the blood is otherwise referred to as "spilling ketones."

Do not mistake ketosis for ketoacidosis. Ketosis a natural and often healthy body process. Ketoacidosis is a life-threatening scenario often experienced by diabetics due to insulin malfunction, hyperglycemia, and simultaneous buildup of acids in the blood. This is caused by a genetic defect, disease, and diabetes, particularly poor diabetes management, poor compliance, or noncompliance. If you're diabetic or suspect you may have diabetes, then consult with your doctor before going on any new diet, exercise, or weight loss program.

Since ketosis means your body is using ketone bodies as fuel and not glucose from your diet, then another process called gluconeogenesis will kick in if your body and brain needs glucose.

Gluconeogenesis is when the brain or other body tissues require glucose for metabolism and function. When you're in a state of carb depletion or ketosis and your body cannot function on using body fat and ketone bodies alone for maintaining body processes, then protein from your diet will be converted into glucose.

You see, the body is very efficient. At all times it seeks balance, so it is able to manifest glucose from protein and ketone bodies from body fat. Of course, for the purpose of your weight loss journey, the goal is to burn off body fat—not protein or lean body mass—for energy, so your strategy to maintain lean body mass and avoid converting protein from your diet to glucose is to consume enough calories of high BV proteins to maintain a positive nitrogen balance, which will keep you in an anabolic state.

The day you begin carb depleting, your glucose-starved body is forced to pull from glycogen storage. Your body will convert glycogen to glucose and use it for necessary body functions, a process called ***glycogenolysis***. When glycogen is depleted from the body's muscle cells, then comes the depletion of liver glycogen. When all muscle and liver glycogen has been metabolized, the body is forced to start pulling from body fat to fuel body functions and work.

Body fat is converted into fatty acids and glycerol through lipolysis.

Lipolysis is the process of burning off adipose tissue, the internal cannibalism of your own body fat, otherwise known as diet-induced thermogenesis. Simply put, it's weight loss by incinerating body fat from your butt, batwings, love handles, double chin, and all the other flabby areas.

Doesn't this sound fantastic? Carb depletion begins the fat-burning process. When glycogen depletion has occurred through depleting carbs, you reach ketosis, which begins the process of incinerating body fat.

The EXERLEAN goal is not to remain *in* ketosis but just *out of* ketosis, to avoid the negative effects of catabolism or starvation and at the same time avoid glycogen storage or replenishment. The goal, when you've achieved glycogen depletion, is to then consume enough high-BV protein and low-fat, low-GI, nonprotein foods to stay out of ketosis. Actually, you'll be hovering just out of ketosis, reaping the benefits of fat burning while preventing the metabolism of lean muscle tissue. This is the State. For most people, it will take three or four days; we'll get to your specific timing later in the chapter.

Step Two: Protein Loading

Days 3 or 4 through 11 or 12

Goal: Promote an anabolic environment in the body by maintaining a positive nitrogen state during carb and calorie restriction. Gluconeogenesis is the backup glucose plan.

This process involves eating just enough low-glycemic carbohydrates to hover just out of a ketosis state. To remain in a positive nitrogen state, which preserves lean body tissue during fasting, you need to provide your body with a continuous stream of protein throughout the day. If you're carb depleting or in a low-GI-carb environment, then protein loading will provide enough protein to heal your body and prevent it from burning muscle instead of fat. And if you need energy, then gluconeogenesis will provide glucose as fuel for your brain and body when necessary. Step two, otherwise referred to as *protein loading*, is when you will burn the most body fat. By maintaining anabolism and a positive nitrogen state during a low-carbohydrate diet, and finally benefiting from lipolysis, you'll incinerate body fat.

Being in this state will promote burning off body fat even without restricting calories below your BMR. Because you are in a glycogen-depleted state, you are in a sense hollow, ready to be filled. In the State, your body must fill up the hollow spaces before it will begin storing fat again. Add to that, eating very low carb and nonfat makes it impossible to fill the hollow back up or add fat back. Because the body remains hollow, and you are eating low- or nonfat low-GI carbs in small enough quantity to remain just out of ketosis, your body is forced to annihilate its fat sacks for energy in the metabolic pathway. Yeah, you are protein loading, but the protein sources you are consuming are low or nonfat, plus protein is the last thing the body wants to convert to fat because it is so valuable to the body as a building block and healer of the body. Protein is also a security blanket for the brain in a low-carb state by providing it glucose through gluconeogenesis.

Now add in calorie restriction as necessary to turn up the dial on the fat-burning furnace without burning muscle and without adding fat back. Adding a calorie deficit to your BMR while in the State gets the thermogenic pathways fired up. Finally add exercise, weight training, and hyperactive ADL (activities of daily living) for the ultimate phase of body fat incineration.

Picture a big fold of cold hard butter sitting in a cold skillet. Turn up the dial to heat up the skillet, and next thing you know, that butter is spattering and smokin' in a red-hot iron skillet. In the State, the butter is your body fat, the dial is your blood chemistry dialed into perfection, and the red-hot skillet is your metabolism. Say hello to your total body fat incinerator.

Yeah, baby!

Here's a quick summary of step two:

Carb depletion forces other energy pathways, leading to **glycogen depletion**.

A state of glycogen depletion forces other energy pathways, leading to **lipolysis, or fat burning**.

A positive nitrogen state through protein loading promotes anabolism, or **muscle growth**.

Body fat is being used for your main energy supply, and if glucose is needed for your brain or other body functions, **gluconeogenesis**, or conversion of protein from your diet to glucose, will ensue.

Weight training, other exercise, work, and hyperactivity promote anabolism, endorphin release, and **metabolism of body fat**.

You are now a body fat–burning, fat-ass incinerating, muscle-building machine.

Hello, new you.

Badass you.

Future you is on the horizon.

Step Three: Carb Loading/Glycogen Refeeding

Days 12 or 13 through 14

Goal: Replenish glycogen stores and keep the body guessing with abrupt variation through low-GI carb loading, in periodic short cycles of one to three days. (One to two days is preferred as a third day of carbing up can be overkill and get you fatter.) Through experience and time, you will learn to listen to your body, take into consideration your weight loss or gain, including what process or format of the algorithm is working best for you, and develop a pattern of executing what is successful for your unique body.

When on a specific diet regimen, calorie-deficit program, or macro-nutrient-restriction program for long enough, the body, as efficient as it is, will adapt to the state of fasting by lowering your BMR. You can prevent this undesirable result by abruptly changing your diet through carb loading, or refeeding. Carb loading is specific to carbohydrates, and refeeding refers to consuming all macros to refuel a void. From here on, we will be mostly referring to the loading or refeeding phase as carb loading because the last thing you want to do is load fat, and you don't need to load protein during the carb-loading phase as you just finished twelve days getting through steps one and two, which included carb depletion and then protein loading, fat depletion, and minimal low-GI carb intake.

Carb loading is unusual to the body after glycogen depletion in step one and then low-carb restriction during step two. Switching suddenly from using body fat for energy back to glucose will reverse the metabolic process. The extra glucose not used for energy will be used to replenish muscle cell and liver glycogen stores. You have been hollow for the last seven days, and now you're filling yourself with muscle glycogen, nutrient replenishment, and energy. It's like hitting the reset button on the whole dang process and then starting over again, except this time you are primed to dominate the process. During carb loading, you will also notice improved overall athletic and physical performance while weight training, exercising, and performing ADL. This will be similar to the benefits an athlete receives from carb loading before an event.

Again, it is important to not over-carb. Over-carbing can lead to spillover of excess calories back into your body fat stores. This is an undesirable outcome, as you just worked so hard to eliminate the same body fat during the fasting cycle.

There are two ways to prevent spillover:

Load low-glycemic carbs only.

Keep calorie consumption to just over BMR. No indulgence, gluttony, or cheating. When in doubt, under-carb.

The process of carb depleting; then low-GI carb, nonfat, high-BV protein loading; and then low-GI carb loading increases your chances of anabolism and prevents your body from accommodating to your diet. By creating extreme variation in macronutrients, fasting, loading, and calorie consumption, you can create an anabolic or growth state in your body and return a crashed metabolic rate back to normal, even raising your BMR over time. This process helps keep your body guessing. When the carb-loading or refeeding cycle is completed, your body is ready for another bout of carbohydrate and glycogen depletion by restarting the State algorithm at step one.

You'll repeat this two-week cycle indefinitely until you have achieved your goal of a lean, ripped body, or whatever you decide is your goal. As long as you continue this process, body fat will keep melting off. As you stick with the EXERLEAN State, you will start to notice trends in your body's response. As you gain a firm grasp of how your body is responding, you can modify the days of each stage to better suit which ones burn body fat at the fastest clip. But this takes many, many months, up to years, and only through following a disciplined regime and keeping track of your results, recording them, and looking back on the data can you make an objective move for change. This is an area of your transformation where journaling is necessary.

You should not go just by feeling but by *subjective* feeling and *objective* data—BMI, body fat percentage, body weight, and observable changes. So for the short term, it is best to stick with the program as it is laid out and modify only if you need to for physical or mental health reasons. For some people, four days of carb depletion is not enough, and for some, two days may achieve the goal of overall glycogen depletion. This is especially so if during the two days of carb depletion you are engaged in heavy weight training and/or cardio.

Step two should not be shortened; if anything, it should be lengthened if the carb-depletion or carb-loading phases are shortened, overall maintaining a two-week cycle. As the program is laid out, you start with four days of carb depletion, followed by eight days of protein loading, followed by two days of carb loading. If you notice you get better results carb depleting for three days and carb loading for three days, your protein loading will be eight days to make a fourteen-day cycle. If you carb deplete four days and carb load one day, you have a nine-day protein-loading phase. Never go less than eight days for the protein-loading phase, never more than four days for carb depletion, and never less than one day, but not more than three, for carb loading. Then repeat. In the beginning and until you're confident in your changes, don't modify the program.

A Deeper Look at Each Step of the State

Let's look at the three stages in this body fat incineration algorithm, the State, and clarify exactly what you need to do step-by-step, including sample meal plans.

Step #1: glycogen depletion. In the first step of the fourteen-day cycle, the goal is total muscle cell and liver glycogen expenditure. Glycogen or carb depletion simply means that you eat zero carbohydrates for two to four days. By eating only protein sources, you force your body to use up all its glycogen stores, eventually reaching a state of ketosis. For example, you could eat lean chicken breasts cooked in a light amount of olive oil for four days straight. Ketosis is typically reached around days two to four of carb depletion.

Carb depletion is technically simple but mentally and sometimes emotionally very difficult. The first time a person goes through carb depletion is the hardest. In carb depletion, you feel true deprivation and a get a glimpse into the feelings of a starving person. The funny thing, though, is you're hardly that bad off during carb depletion because you're consuming more than enough calories to sustain life through the protein sources you are consuming and the body fat you may also be burning.

Protein is a luxury in third-world countries, and you're going to be eating a lot of it. Lucky you, really! And don't forget that if you have obvious body fat, you're definitely not starving in a carb-depleted or calorie-deprived state . . . that's food in them there thunder thighs, bat wings, double chins, chubby cheeks, love handles, and potbellies.

In carb depletion, your brain is instantly not receiving the easy sweet-blood glucose it is accustomed to, which triggers many different neurotransmitter, hormonal, and chemical processes. Restricted of glucose, these chemical pathways trigger hunger pangs, stress, and commonly, fatigue.

When you start calorie restriction and macronutrient deprivation through dieting, you're attempting to take control of your body weight and create change. The problem is that no matter what your weight is, your body has established a set point. A set point is when your body has become accustomed to a certain calorie amount and type of food consumption coupled with your body composition and weight. The ingredients of your set point stake a claim through neuronal mapping in your brain. Your set point is established to whatever status you are typically in, whether morbidly obese, obese, overweight, average, skinny fat, skinny lean, or even muscular lean, bulky muscular, or athletic. When you deviate from whatever your body, under your brain's control, has established as your set point, then your brain will sense this deviation and send out hormones that trigger a return to the set point. If you're trying to gain weight, your body will try to decrease consumption by making you feel full (called satiety). If you're losing weight, your body will send out signals telling itself to consume more by making you feel hungry.

What! **you're saying.** *My body is going to be fighting against me?*
Yup! Every step of the way.

Your body is going to be doing everything it biologically can to counteract your sacrifice of working to burn body fat and lose unhealthy weight. Your body cannot physically make you do anything, like cheat on your diet, but it does have some intense mind-altering hormones in its arsenal—namely leptin and ghrelin—and the ability to release them to coerce you into doing the dirty work for it.

Leptin is an important hormone your body fat tissue releases to get you to stop eating. It is an appetite suppressant, a satiety weapon. See, your body wants to prevent you from losing weight and gaining weight. When your blood sugars are up or your stomach is full, leptin is released to get you to feel full and quit eating. So, for obese people, leptin is a good thing, right? The more body fat you have, the more leptin is released, which is even better, right? Not so. Fat people release so much leptin and then continue to overeat, ignoring the feeling of satiety . . .

the reason for getting fat in the first place, so their bodies get desensitized to the mild-altering effects of leptin, which is trying to convince them to stop eating. In a way, by overeating in the presence of leptin, your biological set point and your brain establish that being full or having high blood sugar in the presence of leptin is normal. Therefore, that feeling of satiety with eating is diminished, or the bar is set pretty high to finally feel full or satisfied.

Since leptin is not helping an obese person feel satisfied, the obese person who wants to lose weight needs to be cognitively, mentally, and emotionally aware (thoughts, mindset, and soul power) of calorie intake and portion control to restrict them. Because their body's natural defense, the leptin pathway, has been damaged, they have to take full control of what, when, and how much they eat to win the fight against their own body wanting to stay fat or even get fatter.

Research has shown that leptin plays a role in metabolism through the adrenal and thyroid pathways that influence muscle energy usage. Some studies show that reducing leptin can lower a person's metabolism, making it more difficult to lose weight, and contrary, leptin supplementation or increased leptin levels may improve the metabolic pathway and promote weight loss. Leptin is not available as an over-the-counter or prescription supplement as of 2020. Studies continue to determine the safety, effectiveness, and application of leptin in the fight against the global obesity epidemic.

The point here is that as you become obese and remain obese, and as your body and brain become desensitized to leptin, the satiety hormone and also a hormone linked to helping increase metabolism, your body establishes obesity as the normal set point. Then when you diet to lose weight, that weight loss will trigger hunger and a drive to eat and return to your set point. So no matter how much weight you lose, let's say 150 pounds, your body will still drive you through chemical and hormonal pathways ordering a return to your original set point. It seems unfair that an obese person has to work harder to lose weight and work just as hard to remain at the new lower weight. This is why obese people who lose a ton of weight have a hard time keeping it off and eventually return to their fat selves. The fact is, gaining weight is preventable. The problem is that dieters give in to their bodies' signals to return to their old set points and their fat selves. All fatback cases are because people stop eating restrictively and return to old eating and behavior habits filled with calorie-dense, high-glycemic, low-protein, high-fat, hyperpalatable foods with low nutritional value and at the same time stop routine exercise.

In this program, it is imperative that you remain vigilant in the restrictive diet you become accustomed to for the long term to keep the weight off, get even leaner, and with discipline and hard work, reset your brain and your body's set point to the new lower weight and lean you. This will happen, but it takes a long time. It took you years to establish your fat set point and desensitize yourself to leptin, and it will likely take you years to establish your low weight and lean set point, and to again benefit from leptin's signals that help you feel full after eating and maximize your metabolism to boot.

This will happen if you remain strong, focused, and in control of your body. You can do this! You choose what thoughts you have, you conjure ideas, and you alone take action and execute what you do in this short life. You must constantly fight against your brain's basic drive to avoid change. Through diligence and perseverance, you will get lean, stay lean, and reset your brain, set point, hormones, and chemicals to accommodate to the new, healthy you. At that point, things will get easier, and maintaining your healthy body will feel normal.

The second strong hormone your body uses to maintain its set point is ghrelin.

Unlike leptin, which triggers satiety when eating, *ghrelin* does the opposite. Ghrelin is a hormone that is released to make you feel hungry and feel a drive to eat. You recall that leptin is a hormone released by fat cells to convince you to stop eating. Ghrelin is release by the stomach and gastrointestinal (GI) tract to convince you to start eating. When your stomach is empty or you have low blood sugar, ghrelin is secreted to signal the brain to make you feel hungry and send you seeking out food. This is what happens when you first start a diet. The bad part here is you can't eat because you're trying to burn body fat. To make it worse, you are addicted to antidiet foods that will only sabotage your weight loss efforts.

Food and poor eating habits can be as addictive as drugs, alcohol, gambling, and sex because they piggyback on the same reward-oriented neural and chemical pathways in the brain. That's especially true for addictive foods referred to as hyperpalatable foods, which have intense sweet and salty flavors piggybacked with fat saturation. People get addicted to foods that are salty, sweet, and fatty, leading to overeating as they try to satisfy cravings and continue receiving the reward benefit, which is pleasure. This process leads to dependency on hyperpalatable foods, which leads to loss of control and failure to remain at a healthy weight. Next thing you know, you're fat.

Now add the addiction of hyperpalatable foods in a chronic overeater to the desensitization of the satiety hormone leptin and, to top it off when trying to lose weight, the hunger-trigger hormone ghrelin kicking into high gear, you're left addicted to the worst kinds of foods, without feeling satisfied and yet with hunger pangs like a starving lion muzzled in a field of fat lambs.

Hyperpalatable food addiction is curable through persistent restriction, which leads to habit change and with it less desire to eat those foods. You can conquer desensitization to leptin by staying diligent in maintaining small portion sizes and not overeating. When you diet, you're restricting food consumption so you can lose weight. As soon as you start carb depleting, the mechanisms to trigger self-feeding kick in.

Remember this: when you are eating restrictively and forcing your body to burn body fat for energy, you're going to feel a strong drive to eat hyperpalatable foods. Hunger pangs will kick in and you may feel like you're starving, but you're not!

The extreme hunger you feel when engaging in a new diet, especially during the first month, is not because you are starving but because your metabolic set point is off and *ghrelin is a yellin'*.

Stay focused. You are not starving in carb depletion or calorie restriction as long as you are protein loading and consuming enough low-GI carbs to hover just out of ketosis. You are forcing your body to eat its own body fat for energy. Unless you are already lean and lightweight, you have plenty of body fat for fuel to burn. Keep pushing forward. Stay mentally strong. Focus intensely on the prize. In this process, you will establish a new set point. Things will get easier.

Why on earth would anyone put themselves purposefully through the process of carb and calorie restriction, which for many dieters results in feeling bad? Well, think about it this way . . . only through sacrifice, hardship, and faith do the most miraculous things happen in life. Through work, struggle, and purpose, we persevere and conquer our most seemingly unattainable dreams. Any suffering you feel during the short blips of carb depletion and calorie restriction is nothing compared to twenty-four hours a day of decreased quality of life you will be dealing with at some point due to obesity. On the contrary, the benefits of achieving a lean, strong, and healthy physique far outweigh the work, discipline, and sacrifices it takes to get there.

Glycogen depletion, calorie restriction, and protein loading work together to move your body into a maximal state of body fat incineration. The goal is to burn body fat at a maximal rate to achieve a lean body, then maintain it for the rest of your life. We are not going to waste your valuable time engaging in a lesser process or program that will likely never achieve results fast enough to keep you motivated and excited about future you. If you have a choice—and you do—would you like to drive a Lamborghini or the Griswolds' woody to the finish line, where your beautiful lean and healthy physique awaits? EXERLEAN is the Lamborghini that will take you to the finish line first. You must keep faith in yourself, remain disciplined, and do the necessary work to earn the physique of your dreams.

From day one of carb depletion, you will need to monitor your body for ketosis. To do this, you use ketosis test strips, which are easily available online or at your local pharmacy. Within seconds of dipping a strip in your urine stream, you will know if you are in ketosis. It is highly unlikely you will be even close to ketosis until the end of step one—day two, three, or four depending on your unique physique and exercise level.

When you reach ketosis, meaning you start spilling ketones into your urine, then it is time to begin step two of the EXERLEAN algorithm. This will usually happen on day three or four of carb depletion, and you will know by the color-coded ketosis test strips. If you need to remain in carb depletion because you have not entered ketosis yet and need more energy for ADL and exercise, then add fat to your diet by supplementing with fish oil, omegas, conjugated linoleic acid (CLA), or yolk in eggs, or by cooking your meats in olive, canola, sesame, or peanut oil.

Nuts and nut butters can be good energy sources during dieting and are usually low carb. They are poor protein sources, however, because they are low on the biological value scale. They have healthy fats and anti-inflammatory properties but are not included in the EXERLEAN fat-burning algorithm because they are highly addictive. Overconsuming them will derail your progress and potentially make you fatter. Maybe down the road on your weight loss journey after you have mastered your body and have adopted new eating habits, you can incorporate nuts and nut butters into your diet, but not now, not when you are weak-minded and addicted to hyperpalatable foods. You do not need to add to the already difficult level of discipline. Nuts are healthy in small amounts and can be incorporated in a maintenance phase, where weight loss and fat burning is no longer the goal.

Aside from nuts, do not consume dairy products during step one. There are too many sugars and carbs in dairy products for carb depleting, although low-carb, low-fat, dairy protein sources can be used in steps two and three.

Good high-BV protein sources during carb depletion are eggs and egg whites, chicken, turkey, fish, buffalo, game, beef, and lean pork. (No soybeans for carb depleting. Remember, soybeans are a carbohydrate source.) If you can't eat meat, eggs, or fish for some reason, then soy protein isolate, whey protein, or calcium caseinate are alternatives.

During carb depletion, you should try to get protein calories from food sources only. Meaning during these two to four days, it is best for liquid calories to come from protein shakes. Again, avoid protein shakes when the goal is glycogen depletion since liquid protein is easier for the body to use in gluconeogenesis to supply itself with glucose—and we don't want glucose at this point. In this step of the game, the focus is on carb depletion and not protein loading. Although you're eating mostly protein, the end goal is glycogen depletion and achieving a state of ketosis. At that point the stage is set to begin the long haul of fat burning and muscle building.

To sum up step #1:

- No carbs.
- Low fat and added healthy fat and oils as needed for energy.
- High BV protein only and no liquid proteins.
- Hydration only through water and 0-calorie drinks like unsweetened coffee, tea, and artificial and naturally flavored drinks.
- Ketosis test strips to monitor for ketosis. If entering ketosis/spilling ketones, initiate step two.

Example day in step #1:
Food prep:
Skillet-fried chicken

- Fry 6 6-ounce lean chicken breasts in 2 tablespoons olive oil.
- Add seasoning and brewer's yeast to taste (optional—increasing sodium during carb depletion helps keep muscles full for workouts).

Nutrition (per breast): 7.1 grams fat (2.6 chicken fat + 4.5 olive oil), 0 carbs, 40 grams protein, 224 calories

Meal schedule:

- **6:00 a.m.**—1 breast
- **9:00 a.m.**—1 breast
- **Noon**—1 breast
- **3:00 p.m.**—1 breast
- **6:00 p.m.**—1 breast
- **9:00 p.m.**—1 breast
- **Before bed/sometime in evening:** Test urine for ketones using ketosis test strips. (If at the end of day two, three, or four you are spilling ketones, initiate step two.)
- Go to bed and get adequate sleep (fasted sleep).
- Repeat at 6:00 a.m. on days two, three, and four.

Total daily calories: 1,344

Total protein: 240 grams (4 calories a gram for protein)

Total fat: 42.6 grams (9 calories a gram for fat)

This example looks like a lot of calories and food, but it is not. This is actually a low-calorie scenario as far as consumption.

Do not forget to include calories from burning off glycogen and body fat!

What? Nobody does this! Well, I do. In the grand scheme of dieting and weight loss, the focus is always on oral consumption of food and calories. Why does the diet industry leave out all the other calories the body consumes from glycogen and body fat? This is food too and should be accounted for. In fact, isn't internal consumption of your body fat the whole point?

In reality:

1,344 consumed calories
+ calories from burning off glycogen
<u>+ calories from metabolizing body fat</u>
you're fine here, definitely not starving

Do not worry about not eating enough. Worry about eating too much. Shit, look around you! The last thing the majority of us need to do is worry about not eating enough.

Now, there is no way to know how many grams of glycogen or body fat is actually metabolized at any given time. This is not actually quantifiable. But it is a fact that if you are in a calorie-deficit state, then the body needs to replace the missing calories, which it does by breaking down glycogen and then body fat. Remember this: if you start to worry about not consuming enough calories, there are calories you are burning that you cannot see and did not eat.

When ketosis is reached, move on to step two.

Step #2: protein loading. Step two is the maintenance of a low-carb state. Glycogen depletion in step one sets the stage. Step two first bumps you out of ketosis and then keeps you hovering just out of it, which is the maximal state of body fat obliteration. Then maintain this state by keeping low-GI carbs high enough to hover out of ketosis but not too high to prevent the process of glycogen replenishment. In this stage of the game, your body is going to be forced to consume its own fat through the thermogenic pathway. This step can be maintained indefinitely because you're not in ketosis, and you're eating plenty of protein to maintain a positive nitrogen state and enough calories to function, then add in all the extra calories from consuming your own body fat for energy. You're just fine here. More than fine, in fact—your body is likely and finally thriving.

When dieting restrictively, it is vital to stay out of the catabolic pathway. You can do this by eating enough or more than enough protein to stay in a positive nitrogen state. In addition, you are also consuming low-GI carbs and healthy fats, preventing your body from entering ketosis. Low-GI carb consumption needs to be high enough to stay out of ketosis but low enough to prevent glycogen replenishment. The fat calories in lean meat will help provide fuel for ADL. The remainder of the body's energy needs will come from metabolizing your body fat. *Yes!* Bye-bye, body fat.

Figuring out how many grams a day of low-GI carbs you need to consume during step two is a mathematical and scientific process. You will pretty much figure this out during each step of the algorithm. From day one of step one, you will be monitoring your body for ketosis. During step two, you will be testing your urine for ketones and adding low-GI carbs until you're no longer spilling ketones. When you achieve this point, the state of fat burning is at its best. You're hovering just out of ketosis and anabolism through protein loading.

Protein loading means consuming 1.5 to 4 grams of protein per pound of lean body mass. Every person is built differently as far as height, weight, shape, metabolism, and genetics. Each person needs to adapt this program to their unique status. Notice I said to eat enough protein based on your lean body mass. This is important to remember because you do not eat according to your whole body weight or scale weight, which includes body fat. If you base your daily calories on what the scale says, you will be overconsuming and get fatter. For example, if you're a 200-pound obese and deconditioned female, you're likely around 40 percent body fat with an actual lean body mass of around 119 pounds hidden under all that body fat.

Knowing that, you should not base your resting metabolic rate on 200 pounds but on 119 pounds. Your resting metabolic rate is based on lean mass, not fat. You need to eat more than enough protein for your *lean* body mass to survive being cannibalized by thermogenesis. To do this, you need to consume enough protein to beat the daily caloric requirements of your resting metabolic rate. From there, your body will use the fat from protein sources and the low-GI carbs as energy for ADL, IADL, work, and exercise. After using any fat and carbs from food, which is calorie restricted, your body is forced to get the remainder of needed energy from its fat stores.

Good high-BV protein sources during step two on a BV scale where a whole egg equals 100 are:

- Whey protein (96–159)
- Chicken (94)

- Fish (76)
- Buffalo
- Game meat
- Beef (80)
- Pork
- Calcium caseinate (77)
- Nonfat cottage cheese
- Nonfat hard cheeses
- Whole eggs and whites (100)

Good *low-GI carbohydrate* sources during step two on a GI scale of 1–100 are:

- Beans/hummus (6–40)
- Oats (55)
- Most brans (30–50)
- Yams, boiled with skin thirty minutes (35–46)
- Sweet potatoes, boiled with skin thirty minutes (40–46)
- Converted rice (38)
- Barley (25)
- Nonstarchy vegetables (10–47)

To sum up step #2:

- High protein/protein loading with high BV only.
- Fibrous vegetable loading (nonstarchy only).
- Low carbs/enough to remain just out of ketosis/restricted to low-GI carbs.
- Low fat and added healthy fat and oils as needed for energy.
- Hydration only through water and 0-calorie drinks like unsweetened coffee, tea, and artificially flavored drinks.
- Ketosis test strips to monitor for ketosis; if entering ketosis, increase grams of low-GI carbs until out of ketosis.

Example day in step #2:

Food prep:

Skillet-fried chicken

- Fry 3 6-ounce lean chicken breasts in 2 tablespoons olive oil.

- Add seasoning like soy sauce, hot sauce, or another sodium product and brewer's yeast to taste (optional).

Nutrition (per breast): 7.1 grams fat (2.6 chicken fat + 4.5 olive oil), 0 carbs, 40 grams protein, 224 calories

Mixed vegetables, frozen (peas, carrots, corn, and green beans)

- Heat according to directions or as applicable.

Nutrition (1 cup): 0 grams fat, 14 grams carbs, 89 calories

Black beans, boiled, frozen, or canned

- Heat or serve according to directions.

Nutrition (1/3 cup): 0.3 grams fat, 13.5 grams carbs, 5 grams protein, 75 calories

Whey protein powder

- Mix 2 scoops with water in a shaker cup.

Nutrition (2 scoops): 2 grams fat, 4 grams carbs, 48 grams protein, 220 calories

Meal schedule:

- **6:00 a.m.**—1 chicken breast, 1 cup mixed vegetables, 1/3 cup black beans
- **9:00 a.m.**—2 scoops whey protein and water
- **Noon**—1 chicken breast, 1 cup mixed vegetables, 1/3 cup black beans
- **3:00 p.m.**—2 scoops whey protein and water
- **6:00 p.m.**—1 chicken breast, 1 cup mixed vegetables
- **9:00 p.m.**—2 scoops whey protein and water
- **Before bed/sometime in evening:** Test urine for ketones using ketosis test strips.
- Go to bed and get adequate sleep (fasted sleep).
- Repeat at 6:00 a.m. daily for seven to ten days depending on days in step one. Then initiate step three.

Total daily food: 18 ounces chicken, 3 cups mixed vegetables, 2/3 cup black beans, 6 scoops whey protein powder with water, water/coffee/tea/0-calorie drinks

Total daily calories: 1,749 (adjust to be 500–750 under BMR by adding or subtracting to protein sources, not carbs, unless spilling ketones, in which case increase grams of complex carbs until just out of ketosis)

Total protein: 274 grams

Total carbs: 81 grams

Total fat: 27.9 grams consumed, plus amount of body fat metabolized

Finally, let's detail how to carb load in step three.

Step #3: carb loading/glycogen refeeding. When you finalize step two in day twelve or thirteen, it is time to shift gears during days thirteen or fourteen and change your diet to promote anabolism, glycogen replenishment, and fuel for workouts. Step one is no carb, step two is low carb, and now step three is high carb, then it's back to step one. This continuous cycle of abrupt changes in macronutrient restriction and loading promotes anabolism, not as in growth by fat storage but by muscle growth, lean mass preservation, and the promotion of fat burning. At this stage in the game, your body has been through carb depletion, then kept in a state of glycogen depletion through low-carb dieting and workouts, so by day twelve of restriction, your body is hollow, primed for refueling and replenishment. It is yearning for carbs and calories for workout energy, glycogen replenishment, and feeling satiety.

In step three, you can worry less about overconsumption and getting fatter, focusing instead on specific refueling tactics that will allow anabolism and glycogen replenishment. You are in a rare state when any calories over your total daily energy expenditure (TDEE) are less likely to be converted to body fat and more likely to be used for energy and glycogen storage.

In step three, you can stop rote cardio to allow or promote glycogen storage. However, it will help to get in heavy low-repetition weight training sessions each day to maximize using the extra fuel and achieve a maximal muscle pump in the major muscle groups. With extra carbs in your bloodstream, your body will be storing glucose as glycogen and expend some of that glucose and glycogen during weight training for workout fuel and muscle hypertrophy, or pump. In steps one and two, you can achieve a good muscle pump through sodium loading and hydration, but you have to time this perfectly. Overall, it is difficult to achieve a muscle pump in steps one and two due to lack of carbs and glycogen, so it is in your best interest to use the carb-loading phase to replenish muscle glycogen and master the muscle pump so you can push against heavy resistance. This process promotes anabolism, or growth of lean body mass, which boosts your metabolism and prevents your muscles from accommodating to your diet. Besides, it is going to feel fantastic to push against weights with the muscle pump and energy to back it.

In the two days of carb loading, your goal is not to burn body fat but to gain muscle size through glycogen storage and muscle hypertrophy. You will, however, likely burn body fat due to the anabolic environment and improved exercise threshold with more intense weight training sessions. Your body weight will increase while your body fat percentage will decrease significantly due to the increased lean body mass that occurs with hydration and glycogen storage. Do not be worried about the scale-weight gain during carb loading because it is natural for the body to establish baseline glycogen status in skeletal muscles and the liver, in which every gram of glycogen replenishment requires 3 grams of water.

According to Mike Samuels' article "Glycogen and Weight Loss" at www.livestrong.com, the average body holds about 100 grams of glycogen in the liver and 400 grams in muscle cells. Each gram of glycogen carries with it 3 grams of water. This accounts for 2 to 3 pounds of body weight fluctuation based on lost or gained muscle glycogen and water weight alone. This is why during step one of carb depletion, the body will lose over 2 to 3 pounds rapidly and why during carb loading will again gain 2 to 3 pounds. The body is moving glucose and water in and out of the energy pathways through glycogen storage or release. Because of these body weight fluctuations, which really have nothing to do with more or less body fat, it is better to focus on body weight during step two. Record and pay attention to your body weight during each day of the entire process, but take into account water and glycogen weight fluctuations during carb loading and depletion, and don't get freaked out by the rapid changes. It is normal to lose weight at the onset of carb depletion and gain weight during carb loading. In the long run, you should be losing permanent body weight through reducing body fat storage. Over time, through practice and experience, you will figure out what works best for your body and then adjust calories, carbs, and protein to tune your body into its prime anabolic and fat-burning state.

Carb loading is successfully accomplished using low-glycemic carbohydrates. Only low-glycemic carbohydrates are used in the EXERLEAN program. Recall that hyperglycemia and with it an insulin response is the enemy of fat burning and the result of consuming high-glycemic or too many carbohydrates.

Remember, it is virtually impossible to burn body fat in a hyperglycemic state. Hyperglycemia leads to insulin surges and the inability to burn body fat, and in the long run, to obesity. Low-glycemic carbs have a low blood sugar response, which leads to a minimal insulin release and ultimately sustained energy, energy storage, and other health benefits. The goal during carb loading or refeeding is to jack your metabolism through change, promote anabolism through macronutrient cycling, fuel weight training sessions to promote muscle growth, replenish glycogen stores, and prepare the body for the next phase of carb depletion.

The benefits of carb loading/refeeding include:

1. Jacking your metabolism to prevent a plateau or accommodation to a specific diet
2. Promoting anabolism through intermittent carb cycling
3. Weight training with glucose and glycogen for fuel, which leads to increased workload, intensity, and repriming the glycogen release and storage mechanism
4. Replenishing liver and muscle cell glycogen
5. Preparing the body for another cycle of carb depletion and restriction

To sum up step #3:

1. Low-glycemic carbohydrates.
2. No high-glycemic carbs.
3. Low- or fibrous-carbohydrate content for the last meal of the day to avoid calorie-dense carbs in your belly during sleep.
4. No liquid calories, which prevents rapid digestion and assimilation.
5. Moderate quantities of fibrous vegetables for bulk and for slowing digestion and assimilation.

6. Moderate amounts of high BV protein to promote anabolism and slower digestion.
7. No ketosis test strips during carb loading.

Example day in step #3:
Food prep:
Skillet-fried chicken

- Fry 3 6-ounce lean chicken breasts in 2 tablespoons olive oil.
- Cut in half.
- Add seasoning like soy sauce, hot sauce, or another sodium product and brewer's yeast to taste (optional).

Nutrition (per breast): 7.1 grams fat (2.6 chicken fat + 4.5 olive oil), 0 carbs, 40 grams protein, 224 calories

Mixed vegetables, frozen (peas, carrots, corn, and green beans)

- Heat according to directions or as applicable. Microwaving is quick and easy.

Nutrition (1 cup): 0 grams fat, 14 grams carbs, 89 calories

Black beans, boiled, frozen, or canned

- Heat or serve according to directions.

Nutrition (1/3 cup): 0.3 grams fat, 13.5 grams carbs, 5 grams protein, 75 calories

Meal schedule:

- **6:00 a.m.**—3 ounces chicken breast, 1 cup mixed vegetables, 1 cup black beans
- **9:00 a.m.**—3 ounces chicken breast, 1 cup mixed vegetables, 1 cup black beans
- **Noon**—3 ounces chicken breast, 1 cup mixed vegetables, 1 cup black beans
- **3:00 p.m.**—3 ounces chicken breast, 1 cup mixed vegetables, 1 cup black beans
- **6:00 p.m.**—3 ounces chicken breast, 1 cup mixed vegetables, 1 cup black beans
- **9:00 p.m.**—3 ounces chicken breast, 2 cups mixed vegetables

- Go to bed and get adequate sleep (fasted sleep).
- Repeat at 6:00 a.m. After two days of carb loading, restart the next cycle at step one.

Daily food totals: 18 ounces chicken, 7 cups mixed vegetables, 5 cups black beans, unlimited water/coffee/tea/0-calorie drinks

Total daily calories: 2,420

Total protein: 195 grams (120 high BV, 75 low BV)

Total carbs: 300.5 (202.5 complex carbs, 98 fibrous carbs)

Total fat: 25.8 grams (21.3 from chicken, 4.5 from beans)

After restarting the next cycle at step one, repeat this process over and over until you have reached your future you goals and have maintained future you status for at least one year. The long maintenance phase after you reach future you is to retrain your body and brain to accept future you as the new norm, which requires revamping all metabolic and body weight set points. We will talk more about the maintenance phase and how to transition to maintenance for life in upcoming chapters.

All meal examples listed in this program are kept simple to help you understand and learn the core concepts. Of course, you can vary the type of high BV proteins and low-GI carbs, but your success in maintaining a disciplined diet state will increase by keeping meal prep and planning as simple as possible.

The algorithm for the ultimate state of weight loss and fat burning is simple:

- **Step one:** Carb deplete to achieve glycogen depletion, then ketosis.
- **Step two:** High-BV protein load to maintain a positive nitrogen state, preserving muscle mass during fasting and adding in a light amount of low-GI carbs to bump you just out of ketosis but not to the point of replenishing glycogen stores.
- **Step three:** Low-GI carb load in a short burst to prevent diet accommodation and prepare your body for another bout of carb depletion followed by repeating the three-step algorithm until you achieve your body composition goal.

How you do each of the three steps is much simpler than it seems. In carb loading, the point is to surprise your carb-starved body with an abundance of carbs, which will trigger a metabolic response, reprime your glucose and glycogen mechanisms, replenish glycogen storage, and prepare your body for the next cycle, which you repeat until you're finally lean as hell and feeling like a million bucks!

There are plenty of opportunities in the day to eat high-BV protein sources and low-GI carb sources, work out, engage in fasted cardio, and sleep. Most of the food we consider staples are off limits when the goal is weight loss and treating obesity.

The foods you ate that helped you get overweight or obese will not help you treat it. Any diet program that allows you chocolate frickin' cake is giving you a false narrative that will help you get lean and healthy *never*. The results you will see in diets that allow pizza, cake, cookies, taquitos, or whatever fat-and-carb-combined foods are slow to nonexistant. Just because the fitness model on Instagram can eat desserts all the time doesn't mean that is going to work for you.

The people advertising or embellishing this type of eating all the time are most likely already in great shape, work out often, and have taken their body to a place where some of that kind of shit eating is tolerable short term. If an overweight, obese, or morbidly obese person thinks this freelance eating will work for them to lose body fat weight, they are mistaken. This is delusional. This is a road to frustration and ultimately failure.

Every time a person puts low biological value protein, high glycemic carbs, and fat in their body, they are trading the opportunity to put in high BV, low-GI, and nonfat foods, which in turn will keep blood sugar low, prevent insulin spikes, and prevent obesity. Every time a person puts high-glycemic carbs or too many carbs in their mouth, they will get a high blood sugar response, and then it is impossible for the body to metabolize body fat. Instead, it is encouraged to store glucose in your bloodstream as more body fat. Hello, fatter you! Every time you put carbs in your mouth instead of protein, you take away the opportunity to achieve a positive nitrogen state, which promotes muscle preservation during fasting, adds lean muscle tissue, and increases your basal metabolic rate. Every time you put a high quantity of fat in your mouth, you turn your blood into a sludge-like stream of fatty acids and cholesterol, which leads to cardiovascular disease, arteriosclerosis, plaque buildup, and eventually heart attack, stroke, or death.

To help your body change into a body fat incinerator, you must force it into a state of fat burning, or thermogenesis. This can*not* be done with chocolate and pizza . . . sorry!

We humans have made eating so frickin' complicated that the mere idea of dieting is overwhelming. Eat this, eat that, don't eat it, eat all of it, in these proportions, during these times—the millions of options, unlimited tastes, textures, and opportunities, and people to eat with is staggering. It's almost paralyzing when it comes to the journey of weight loss, especially when you're initiating a diet and exercise plan.

The key to your successful weight loss in this environment is simplicity, discipline, more simplicity, more discipline, avoidance of negative external forces—especially negative people, fuck the naysayers—then some more simplicity and discipline. This shit is simple if you let it be. *EXERLEAN* has laid out key concepts, steps, rules, and strategies to help you turn your body into a fat-burning incinerator, build up your metabolism, and achieve your best health ever . . . future you. You just need to keep the process simple. Every day simple. Every meal plan simple. Meal preparation simple. This may involve eating the same food choices every meal, every day, for weeks and months with the goal of establishing a baseline, adopting it, loving it, and living it.

After living at baseline for a few months, anything you add for variety and flavor will be much more rewarding. For example, after eating chicken breasts as your only meat source for a month, a steak will taste unusually fantastic. Until you have mastered your body and health, keep the process simple, simple, and simpler. Anything you can do to make the whole deal easier will help you stay on track and endure the long journey ahead. Who says that meals and eating must be complicated, vast, and social? Food is a tool. A tool for the body to use as fuel, repair, and maintenance. Change the way you view food, use food, and think about food, and focus on what really matters in life, like love, fun and rewarding experiences, people, productivity and work, sex, and your health.

- Food is a tool used as fuel and as building and repair in the human body.
- Food in itself has zero power at burning fat off your body.
- Food in itself, however, is the only culprit adding fat to your body.
- Your body is a machine.

- Your body needs fuel.
- Your body can burn body fat or food for fuel. Only in the State can the body pull from body fat stores and metabolize it for energy.
- Food can be used as a tool to help your body achieve the State of ultimate fat burning.
- Food can be used to fuel and repair your body and simultaneously support a fat-burning state.

This is EXERLEAN.

At this point, it is vital to cure your overweight or obese status, master your mind and body, adopt restrictive habits and behaviors, and establish a positive social environment around you that will promote and help you maintain awesomeness for the rest of your life.

I've said it before: your life depends on it.

Obesity comes with a shitstorm of negative sequela—chronic complications that are aftereffects of this unhealthy condition—and with it decreased quality of life, which only gets worse with aging. The financial costs of buying high BV proteins, protein powders, veggies, and low-GI carbs is insignificant compared to the costs that obesity will wreak in your life.

Obesity will likely lead to early death, diseases like diabetes and resulting possible amputations, physical disability, and overall diminished quality of life. Health insurance premiums will be higher for future unhealthy obese you. How long will you be able to continue working? Will the negative effects of obesity and aging prevent you from working until your retirement age? Will you become disabled before being able to collect social security and Medicare? Will remaining obese lead to an inability to self-care, the inability to wipe your own ass, dependence on others, and nursing home care? The lifetime costs of obesity are cataclysmic compared to the costs of buying high-quality foods and a gym membership now. Not to mention if you take in mind the sample meal plans listed earlier, they are so affordable you will likely be saving money. Eat lean for every meal, everyday long term and you will save a ton of money. Eating lean helps you cut back on eating larger portions and especially when eating out leading to a lower dining bill. Not only does eating lean help you lose weight, it can also put more money in your wallet in the long run.

Remember Bodinomics and the economy of the human body? Use the cost-benefit analysis to help weigh in on the cost of healthy food versus the cost of obesity. The cost of simplicity versus the cost of complexity/variety. The cost of being sedentary versus the cost of exercising.

- Do the math.
- Follow the rules.

The cost-benefit analysis is full proof. Good always wins. Better choices prevail. You do the right work, and you will attain the right results.

KISS (keep it simple, silly) is a very important concept in your long-term weight loss and health maintenance plan. Eat the same high BV proteins, the same low-GI carbs, and restrict fat until you are lean and healthy. Live at baseline until it feels like the norm, then at that point, which may be months or years down the road, you can add more variety yet remain restricted enough to maintain a lean and healthy body for life.

For life . . .

I can hear it now. The peanut gallery. The naysayers. The politically correct diet experts, fake food news, fake diet gurus, phony fad-diet propaganda, and other bullshit flooding your senses and trying to alter your ability to reason. To give you doubt. To derail you from your mission. Your mission to change yourself for the better. You might hear them all saying:

"Is it unhealthy to eat the same thing every day?"

"What about all the different vitamins, minerals, and stuff the body needs?"

"Is cycling proteins and carbs healthy?"

"Is eating low fat healthy?"

"Is eating a lot of protein healthy?"

"Is carb depleting healthy?"

"Is taking extremes sustainable?"

"Is depriving yourself of life's eating pleasures worth it?"

Blah, blah, blah. Same old shit that is put out there to help you fail in your fat-loss journey. The same old shit that keeps cycling around in air to keep everyone fat, keep everybody down, and prevent you from moving toward something better for yourself.

Being overweight or obese in itself is an extreme, and it took extreme overeating and piss-poor health choices to achieve. You can debate the benefits or negatives of any reputable diet program on earth, but none will ever be as unhealthy as obesity itself. Therefore, what do you have to lose by taking measures that will help treat and prevent obesity? Nothing! You have nothing to lose other than a fat ass and in turn, everything to gain and look forward to in your aging years.

Now is the time to prepare for your future. The choices you make and the work you do now dictate your future circumstances.

Do you look forward to a future of physical ability, of mental and body wellness? Of course you do! The last thing anyone wants is to suffer or live in regret, wishing they would have taken action when they physically could have and should have done the work.

This is your last stand. Time for action before it is too late and the effects of obesity overtake you.

You decide.

You make you.

You are 100 percent responsible for your health, body, and lifestyle choices. Screw the naysayers and negativity that will continue to attempt to surround you like a blanket of stitched cactus barbs.

Ask any professional bodybuilder, athlete, or successful person: when you declare a change and make observable progress, the world around you, including your loved ones—especially loved ones—will become a negative force set on tempting and seducing you into sabotaging yourself and your mission. This is because when you change yourself, it forces those around you to change the way they relate to you, envision you, and interact with you. It's human nature to fight change. To take the path of least resistance.

You must overpower negative external forces. Future you is on the horizon.

The most brilliant experts and every bit of scientific research detail how horrific obesity is to a human being's mortality, yet when it comes to taking action, restricting food, fasting, and doing what is necessary to treat obesity, then all of a sudden . . . negativity.

I'm sure you've heard the proverb, "You can't have your cake and eat it too." Well, "You can't have obesity and health too." The two are opposite forces. You cannot treat obesity without food restriction and physical activity. When your body fat or obesity is gone, then you can say your physique is healthy.

How about focusing on the most important fact! Being overweight and worse off, obese and eating whatever the heck you want is slowly killing you. There is much more research out on the negative effects of eating too many calories, consuming too many carbs, not eating enough protein, and eating too much fat, so the ideas laid out in this book, which if you give them an honest chance, just may help you get in the best shape of your life.

Life is short, and change cannot happen unless you actually change. If you want to be in the 1 percent, you must do what the 1 percent do to get there. This goes for earning riches and success as well as creating a contest winning a lean and healthy physique. If you want to look like the attractive lean people in magazines, movies, and competitions, then you must find out what they do and do it. If you want to get leaner, whether your goals are to compete in a bodybuilding competition or just burn off as much body fat as fast as possible, then your best bet is to do what the people with the best physiques in the world do. I promise you that the 1 percent best are doing, in various methods and tailored to their own personal needs, all or some of the principles and protocols in the EXERLEAN fat-burning algorithm. The 1 percent keep things simple, remain disciplined day after day, get up earlier than everybody else, and work their butts off every day.

You too can achieve your 1 percent.

Let's go through a successful day in the life of Marco in his mission to achieve the State of ultimate body fat incineration. (Don't worry, I haven't forgotten about Jane; to keep things simple, we'll assume from here on out she follows the EXERLEAN program along with Marco.)

Marco is sick and tired of being fat and having low energy, and he is depressed about his predicament. He has decided he wants to take a stand and lose some weight. Little does he know what he is in for when he buys *EXERLEAN* and begins reading. Marco never realized just how bad being obese is to a person's morbidity and, likely sooner than necessary, their mortality. Shaken by what he has read and now feeling the sting of truth, he makes a vow to himself to change his ways. To take everything he has learned and use the EXERLEAN fat-burning protocol to achieve future him. He can visualize his future self and how good he will feel when he makes his dream body a reality.

Marco sets a date and prepares to turn his body into a fat-burning furnace . . . **the State**. He goes to Costco and buys a few bags of frozen boneless skinless chicken breasts, a bag of Optimum Nutrition Gold Standard 100% Whey protein powder, a few bags of stir fry vegetable blend, and a couple of cases of eight-can packs of black beans. For seasoning, he gets a bottle of soy sauce, Bragg Liquid Aminos, a jar of minced garlic, brewer's yeast, Johnny's Seasoned Pepper, and low-sugar salsa. Marco has gathered the foods necessary to embark on his first cycle of steps one, two, and three. Now for *food prep*.

He marinates all the chicken in an olive oil, vinegar, and teriyaki brine. To prepare the chicken, Marco uses his conventional oven to bake the meat thoroughly. Cooking chicken covered in the oven will keep the chicken moist, which makes eating chicken easier. Dry chicken is difficult to eat without condiments or side carbs, and these are not options in step one. The mixed vegetables, black beans, and whey protein do not need any prep since they are ready to use . . . simple! For step one, Marco plans to eat six to seven chicken breasts a day for four days. That is all. This will help him deplete his glycogen stores and enter ketosis. He puts each chicken breast in freezer-quality storage bags or microwave-safe containers and divides his lot into four days.

Next, Marco purchases ketosis test strips at the local pharmacy. A seasoned bodybuilder or other fitness professional can monitor ketones without test strips because they have put thousands of hours into the process and have mastered their bodies. I have mastered my body and am aware of when I am in or close to entering ketosis, and at that point, I make sure by testing for ketones. Some signs of nearing ketosis are sweet-smelling breath, extreme brain drain or mental acuity deficits, and observing or feeling flat, exhausted muscles. You should not try this process without ketosis test strips until you have been through the process many times and experienced how your body responds to carb depletion. When you have mastered your body and are fine-tuned to its status and needs, then you will know by feeling when you are close to entering ketosis. Remember, though, it takes much time and experience to master this process.

Marco also purchases a body weight scale to record his beginning and daily weights to track what is happening to his body. He takes many pictures of his body from different angles with as little clothing on as possible so he can always refer back to where he started on his journey. This is an important step. Without beginning pictures, you will be unable to reference your progress or lack thereof because you will be accustomed to where your body is presently and forget what it once was.

To prepare for step two, the State, Marco plans three food meals and three whey protein shakes a day. Each meal will consist of a chicken breast, 2/3 cup of black beans, and 1 cup of mixed vegetables except for the third meal, which will be carbless to prepare the body for fat burning during sleep . . . *fasted sleep*. For the eight days of step two, which takes him halfway through the cycle, he places twenty-four Tupperware dishes on the counter, three for each day. Sixteen get one chicken breast, 1/3 cup of black beans, and one cup of mixed vegetables. The other eight dishes get one chicken breast, no beans, and one cup of mixed veggies. They all go in the freezer, ready to be pulled out when needed.

If twenty-four meals in the freezer is too much for you, then you need to meal prep more often. I meal prep once a week for seven days' worth of meals, all in the freezer ready to eat or to go.

So far, Marco has completed four days of step one and all food prep for step two, so on day eight, he will prep for the remaining two days of the two-week cycle—step three: two days of carb loading.

Marco plans to consume all food meals and no liquid calories. He is going to prepare ten meals containing 3 ounces of chicken, 1 cup mixed veggies, and 1 cup black beans, then for step three, two evening meals with 3 ounces of chicken and 1 cup mixed veggies. This concludes all his meals for fourteen days. No going out to eat and no cooking except for meal-prep day leaves you with much extra time to put toward the *EXER* in EXERLEAN.

Now that we have thoroughly gone through the process of achieving the State, meal prep, and strategies to avoid failure, we need to talk about weightlifting and fasted cardio.

EXERLEAN's mission is to help you get in the best physical, mental, and emotional state you can possibly achieve. The mission includes both strategic dieting and exercise.

No one can achieve the best possible outcomes of health and wellness without both exercise and diet. Daily exercise and diet throughout your lifespan is vital to thrive in health and wellness, then to maintain that awesomeness indefinitely.

In the fourteen-day cycle, you should make every effort to get in cardio first thing every morning on an empty stomach, taking advantage of the benefits of fasted cardio. If you cannot get cardio in first thing, then anytime you can, you should. Every day you should strive to engage in your ADL, IADL, and work with hyperactivity and ferocity toward productivity to help you burn off extra body fat. Weightlifting each body part once a week is essential. You can weight train one day a week or seven days a week as long as you are getting in each body part at least once a week. The more you split up the body parts, the more days you need at the gym. If you decide to follow my designer workout protocol, Weight Chaining, then you will work out each muscle group once a week in just two days. Chaining is efficient and productive, and it promotes extension in the body, leading to improved posture and functional resting muscle tone. The workouts may be a bit longer, but you have the benefit of five days off to take care of other personal occupations, hobbies, food prep, walks, or other active endeavors.

The main idea here is you need to exercise, and the exercise you need for the rest of your life involves weight training and cardiovascular activity. We went through the benefits of exercise earlier in the book, so you should understand by now that exercise is vital in attaining your maximal state of health, wealth, and wellness.

This concludes the State. We have discussed pretty much everything necessary to understand why we must fight obesity with all our might and engage in a healthstyle that promotes happiness, enjoyment, exercise, and restrictive eating, one that entails deep-seated self-discipline, habit change, self-confidence, and self-control. With this knowledge under your belt, it's time to discuss one of the most controversial yet necessary elements of healthy living: supplements.

CHAPTER 21
Supplementation

IN THIS JOURNEY of self-actualization, health seeking, and physical change, you must take advantage of all the world has to offer to ensure a win. Supplements streamline the process. Supplementation will fill the nutritional voids created by restrictive dieting, work schedules, and other time-crunch dilemmas. The alternative to supplementation is excuses. Excuses ranging from cost, quality, effectiveness, and so on. Cost is not a factor when considering the costs of not doing what is necessary to win your healthy body and achieve a lasting state of wellness in your life. Much research concludes with the positive benefits of nutritional supplementation, plus a plethora of pro athletes, Olympians, professional bodybuilders, trainers, therapists, and doctors can speak on a personal level as to the benefits of supplementation in their personal lives and aiding in successfully maintaining health and wellness.

What is effective is relative to your personal goals and what outcomes you are seeking. Is whey protein powder more effective than egg whites? Maybe, maybe not. What matters is that you are consuming high biological value protein, and if whey protein shakes help you do this, then they are a valuable and effective asset. Not everyone is a stay-at-home person with all the time in the world to food prep, cook, and prepare fresh meals in perpetuity, so for them, supplementation is necessary to maintain the fight against obesity.

EXERLEAN encourages use of the basic supplements like protein powders, amino acids, healthy fats, caffeine, vitamins, and minerals. These natural food products are broken down into powders, pills, and drinks to make consumption easier and more accessible. When it comes to designer supplements, herbs, and other minimally researched nutritional supplements, use at your own caution. EXERLEAN discourages against unknown and under-investigated supplements. That being said, it makes sense to use the food supplements available to help you earn your new lean and healthy body. Future you is on the horizon.

Protein

Protein supplementation is the number one supplement in general. Protein is the most important macronutrient throughout your life. Protein is the *only* nutritional entity that heals and repairs your body, builds it up stronger, and helps prevent disease and disability.

Protein quality is understated in society nowadays with so much focus on vegetables, veganism, and hate of meat. Well, I hate to break it to you, but strict vegan diets done incorrectly are dangerous and in the long term may lead to a lower BMR, muscle wasting/sarcopenia, decreased immunity, decreased strength and power, and possible shorter lifespan. It is obvious that if you starve yourself of protein, your body is going to waste away. Vegetable protein is a low-BV/low-quality protein source and must be consumed in very high amounts to even get an adequate amount of protein, and yet it still remains low biological value. There is only one way a vegan diet can be sustained for you to maintain true physical health, and that is to supplement with soy isolate protein powders throughout the day. And if you're not strict vegan, then whey, egg whites, and casein are high-BV protein options.

Why not soybean burgers and the such instead of soy isolate powder? This is because soybeans are a carbohydrate and high calorie, and if you consume too much, you will be over-carbing and get fatter. Soy isolate powder has little to zero carbs and is a high-BV protein source, which will help support a positive nitrogen state and anabolism on a vegetarian diet. Soy protein isolate in conjunction with soybean foods will be beneficial.

Whey and casein protein powders are straight up high BV protein and when consumed together will give the super high BV of whey with the congealing and slower assimilation quality that comes with casein. Brewer's yeast and soy isolate protein powders have full-spectrum amino acid profiles and great nutritional benefit when taken with high BV whey, casein, and animal proteins.

Recommendations: Whey protein, whey protein isolate, casein, mixed protein blends, egg white powder, brewer's yeast, and soy protein isolate. Take when necessary according to how you feel and/or time since your last consumed protein. Do this in order to maintain a positive nitrogen state, anabolism, and rejuvenation of the body during fasting and exercise. Never skip meals, and use protein supplements liberally to fill necessary gaps in your daily meal plan.

Multivitamins and Minerals

The next most important supplement pair in the EXERLEAN program is multivitamins and minerals. Even if you're not dieting, you should consider these because most foods nowadays are lacking everything necessary for maximal physical, cognitive, and mental health. Vitamin and mineral supplementation is even more beneficial when dieting due to possible lack of variety and fasting, which may create vitamin and mineral deficiencies.

Recommendations: One multivitamin a day, extra vitamin C a day, and additional calcium.

Amino Acids

Amino acids are the building blocks of protein, the most important macronutrient for the body. As we've mentioned, some amino acids cannot be produced by the body and must be consumed in food or through supplementation. Anyone dieting, bodybuilding, or preparing for and engaging in an athletic event may benefit from branched-chain amino acid supplements. There are many brands and supplement companies out there selling amino acid products. Whatever you decide, health experts recommend choosing a high-quality amino acid supplement without stimulants. NO_2 amino acids supplements may help you achieve a killer muscle pump during a weight training session.

Recommendations: Stir 5–10 grams of branched-chain amino acid powder in water or time release in a shaker cup. Consume whenever in a fasting void and during an energy crash, post-workout, or pre-weight training. Take NO_2 supplements before your weight training and cardio sessions to promote blood flow, muscle pump, and nitrogen retention during exercise.

Healthy Fats

Finally, when on a diet, you can supplement with healthy fats to promote necessary hormone, digestion, and metabolic functions. Healthy fats include fish oil, omega fatty acids, CLA (conjugated linoleic acid), MCT oil (medium-chain triglycerides), canola oil, and extra virgin olive oil.

Because people typically don't eat fish often enough, daily fish oil is usually beneficial. CLA and MCT oils can help increase energy and metabolic pathways. Canola and olive oils are great to cook with.

Recommendations: Supplement with fish oil daily, and cook with olive, canola, or peanut oil. Many nonstick sprays made from olive or canola oil can help minimize how much fat you use for cooking, resulting in lower-calorie end products.

There are a plethora of other supplements available, some of which may be great for you and others that may not benefit you at all. I recommend researching the supplement you are interested in trying, reading customer reviews, and looking at the basic science behind the product's claims. When it comes to any herbs, tubers, fungus, roots, or other atypical products, it is important to be aware of any contraindicated outcomes like liver, stomach, heart, and kidney damage. I recommend against cannabis supplementation and alcohol use when on a fat-loss regimen as both have negative results and will hinder your progress. It is well documented that cannabis makes your hunger drive worse, and the last thing you need on a restrictive diet is to be hungrier than is natural and simultaneously less inhibited. Alcohol lowers your testosterone, which is bad for both men and women. Alcohol does not help in any way with fat loss or health and wellness. However, a light beer or glass of wine now and again may help with life enjoyment and could be your biweekly reward for getting shit done.

Do the work. Reap the reward. If you make it through two weeks of the EXERLEAN fat-burning algorithm—the State—then you have earned a light beer or a glass of wine or two before initiating step one for another bout of fasting . . . but no more! Stay focused! Future you is coming. It will be here before you know it so long as you stay on track, stay focused on the prize, and remain true to yourself and this process.

PART 4

Execute & Launch

CHAPTER 22
Putting It All Together

THE FACT REMAINS: seven out of ten adults are overweight, obese, or morbidly obese. These numbers are staggering, an insult to humanity. The Obesiboomer generation is in full effect and in desperate need of an awakening, a movement toward self-awareness, personal responsibility, and action.

Obesity is a self-made affliction putting you at higher risk of an onslaught of obesity-related diseases and looming disability. Knowing at some point that being obese may lead to the inability to wipe your own ass or stand out of a chair without assistance should be enough to trigger self-treatment. The negative effects of obesity on self-care, functional mobility, and quality of life should be a face slap for anyone at risk. Awareness of the negative effects of obesity alone should propel or cattle prod you toward change. If this knowledge does not motivate you or muster the courage to try, then nothing different results. Don't let this be you. Decide for the better.

The first and all subsequent questions, whether you should or shouldn't lose weight, can be contemplated using the laws of Bodinomics and the cost-benefit analysis. When using the cost-benefit analysis to make a decision, you must always choose the heavy-handed, more beneficial decision over the costly one to be successful in life. If a choice has heavy-handed costs over benefits, then the answer for the decision is a no. The same goes for work and fuel. If work, whatever it is, will benefit your life or physical body over the costs, then engage at every opportunity so long as it is a heavy-handed benefit over costs. Fuel—choosing what to eat or not to eat—is the most important time to use the cost-benefit analysis when the goal is to burn off body fat. If the food choice will have more costs than benefits, then do not eat it. If all your food choices are executed using this formula, then you will consume only beneficial foods, resulting inevitably in improved health and wellness.

Exercise is the first half of the EXERLEAN formula. The *EXER* in EXERLEAN. Your best friend in the lifelong battle to win a healthy mind, body, and spirit. Exercise gets your blood flowing. Exercise promotes the release of endorphins and other feel-good chemicals, which course through your veins and stimulate your body and mind. The benefits of exercise are vast and necessary for achieving and then maintaining a life of absolute wellness. Exercise balances out the negative costs of sedentary inaction.

The way you decide to live, move, eat, behave, love, hate, interact, engage, and habituate is the complex art of your healthstyle. Does your healthstyle have a healthy balance of work, play, and sleep? You cannot reap the benefits of work without actually completing the work. Play frees the soul from the clutches of work. You have plenty of time to sleep when you are dead. Don't waste a drop of awake time, and get it all done.

The body needs work. Work keeps your mind and body engaged in an action leading to a productive outcome. Weight-resisted work or manual labor causes reactions in your body that make it grow stronger, instigates healing and balance between different body forces, and fuels the vitality of cellular life. Weight training is the best weapon to use in your fight for maximizing metabolism, gaining muscle mass, and stimulating other positive changes in the body.

EXERLEAN's designer weight training protocol, Chaining, works every muscle group in the body in two days. Chaining promotes extension and aids in the constant fight against gravity. The day you lose the fight against gravity, death is on the horizon.

The yin to balance out weight training's heavy-handed yang is cardiovascular activity. Timed correctly, cardio can be a great fat-burning tool, especially when completed in a fasting state, otherwise referred to as *fasted cardio*. When you've fasted long enough, your blood sugar is low, your glycogen is depleted, and your stomach is empty—a state primed to pull from body fat stores for energy during cardio.

Pain is a natural and necessary sensation in life. Pain can be good or bad. Pain is a signal that you are either injured or worked, the latter being a benefit and the prior a cost. Delayed onset muscle soreness as the result of a weight training or other exercise regimen is good pain. It's your signal of accomplishment and successful treatment to the body.

No pain. No strain. No gain.

This is EXERPAIN! Enjoy it and be happy, for you did the work. You beat resistance.

The obesity battle hinges on the state of your blood. Is your blood too sweet? Cannibalistic? Sludge-like from fat? Spilling ketones? Lacking nitrogen? The ultimate weapon in the arsenal in the war on obesity is to achieve *the State*, the perfect blood chemistry hovering just *out* of ketosis, avoiding the negative catabolic costs of ketosis yet benefiting from the reward of body fat incineration.

The State is reached through a process of carb depletion then carb cycling and strategic protein loading to harness the anabolic benefit of being in a positive nitrogen state, then strategically managing blood glucose through manipulating low-glycemic carbohydrates.

The elite, the 1 percent who are competitive bodybuilders, athletes, wrestlers, MMA fighters, models, dancers, movie stars, and shredded, lean others, know about and use the benefits of being in the State, which contributes to their advantage and ultimately extraordinary success in life.

Now that you know the secret to body fat incineration, what are you going to do?

Contemplate?

Plan?

Prepare?

Execute?

Do the work?

Sacrifice?

Do more work?

Fight against resistance every step of the way?

Reap the rewards of your labor?

Maintain the awesomeness of future you for a lifetime?

"Let's do this!"

The time has come to prepare you for the blastoff, the execution of your journey.

It's action time! To be ready, you must prepare the launchpad. Preparation prevents catastrophic failure during launch. Preparation will help you keep your momentum train moving forward during the beginning phase and into your weight loss and transformation endeavor, when most people fail, quit, crash and burn. You do not want to find yourself lost and scurrying about for answers, tools, supplements, or food after you have already begun. Let us prepare.

CHAPTER 23
Preparation + Execution + Launch!

TO MAKE YOUR transformation as stress-free as possible, preparation is necessary. Before you can enjoy the benefits of dieting and exercise, you must lay the groundwork that facilitates the process. If you want to reap the rewards of exercise and diet, then you're required to do the work. You will never achieve your dream body and healthy life if you don't execute every action necessary to achieve your goals. If you think you can skip the groundwork, then you will fail. The preparation and groundwork facilitate your forward momentum by creating the least restrictive environment during your transformation journey. The work, preparation, organization, and scheduling are the foundation for what is done.

I've mentioned that I believe in having a start date. The start date is the first day of restriction on your two-week cycle. It is when you become 100 percent married to your exercise and diet plan. I don't want you scattered, stressed, or unprepared for the journey ahead. Before you can start, you must have all the right stuff in place.

Where are you going to execute the *EXER* in EXERLEAN? Are you going to complete your fasted cardio and weightlifting at home? If so, do you have an elliptical trainer, treadmill, or other cardio equipment? Do you have free weights or a universal gym, or do you plan on doing all your fasted cardio and weightlifting at a commercial gym? Exercise and weightlifting are necessary engagement during your transformation program. Other than diet, exercise is the only other weapon in your arsenal in the fight to treat and prevent obesity. You will be shooting yourself in the foot if you think you can transform your body and achieve a positive healthstyle without it. So before you make that start date, get a

EXERLEAN: Resolution for the physique transformation of a lifetime.

gym membership, a home gym setup, or some other means to meet the requirements of the *EXER*.

Now consider the *LEAN* in EXERLEAN. What are you going to eat? When are you going to complete food prep for the week? Did you go shopping and load up the freezer with high-BV protein sources and bags of frozen veggies? Is the cupboard full of whey protein powder and a vitamin and mineral supplement? Before your start date and during your program, it is important to remain one step ahead on food prep to make your dieting journey easier. Food prep, cooking, and packaging should all be completed before you need your next meal, which should be ready to eat. If you are running low on protein powder, high-BV protein meats, frozen veggies, and low-GI carb sources, then it is time to hit the grocery store.

Never missing a scheduled meal during a restrictive diet program is just as important, if not more so, as avoiding unplanned calorie consumption.

You eat to live, not vice versa.

I have found that warehouse stores like Costco make everything easier by having a few EXERLEAN-approved choice selections. Bags of lean chicken breasts, lean beef burgers, and many fish options are all high quality and sold in bulk. Costco has huge bags of fibrous veggies in stir-fry mix; a pea, carrot, corn, and green bean mix; a Normandy mix; broccoli; and others that are perfect for your meal plan. For starchy low-GI carbs like yams, sweet potatoes, oats, and rice, any grocery store will suffice. The same goes for healthy cooking oils, fish oil tablets, and other omegas.

Supplements need to be on hand before your start date and then resupplied when necessary to prevent missing a scheduled meal or shake. Protein powder is the number one supplement you need to keep stocked. Shaker mugs are a necessity for getting in all your protein shakes for a day. Protein shakers are available at your local nutrition or supplement store, online, or as supplement company giveaways at bodybuilding competitions.

The best and most convenient deals I've found are at Costco, Walmart online, and Amazon. I usually compare prices on a product between the three, factor in shipping costs, and go with the best deal that will arrive the soonest. I find that Costco is the best place to get whey protein powder, pre-workout stimulants, and amino acids. Chaos Nutrition has some popular workout stimulants, aminos, and other products worth checking out. Walmart online is great for branched-chain amino acids, pre-workout aminos and stimulants, and protein powder. Vitamin and mineral supplements are available at pretty much any major store that sells food. Where you decide to get your protein, aminos, omegas, vitamins, and other supplements doesn't matter as long as you choose high-quality brands.

To store your prepared meals, you obviously need a freezer. Many fitness enthusiasts, including myself, invest in a large freezer to keep frozen protein and veggie sources always within reach. You also need enough freezer-quality containers for a week of meal prep, made of plastic, glass, or whatever toots your fancy. You may not always be a week ahead, but you will find that when you do prepare a week's worth of meals, the whole dieting thing goes much smoother. Food containers are available at department stores, grocery stores, and warehouses like Costco, IKEA, Walmart, and Sam's Club.

Of course, you need to have a way to cook, so ideally you have a stove, oven, and grill to cook your foods and a microwave to nuke your frozen prep meals.

Seasonings and condiments make your food a hell of a lot more palatable. No crazy high-calorie and sugary condiments; go for salt, pepper, cayenne, garlic salt, garlic powder, onion powder, garlic, onions, seasoning salt like Johnny's Seasoning Salt, steak seasoning, Worcestershire, soy sauce, liquid aminos, taco sauce, hot sauce, rooster (sriracha) sauce, salsa, mustard blends, and other low-calorie, low-sugar, nonfat findings.

Everyone needs emergency meals on standby for unforeseen circumstances. For emergency meals that won't throw you off your diet, consider options like jerky made from lean beef, chicken, turkey, or pork; fibrous veggies; and whey protein in a shaker with a water bottle ready to mix. Always have a bag of jerky in your purse, briefcase, car, or work desk, and if you're really feeling ambitious, then pack your small cooler with fresh-cut veggies, a nonfat, low-sugar Greek yogurt, nonfat cottage cheese, or other nonfat, low-carb, low-calorie snacks. Being prepared at all times will prevent catastrophic failure, cheating, and losing your fat-burning state.

Your mission if you so choose to take it is to achieve and then remain in the State of ultimate body fat incineration until you have fully unwrapped your present: future lean and healthy you. This message will self-destruct in five seconds.

If you are really in it to win it . . . and I know you are, then there are more things that will help you monitor, engage, and continue on the path to success. We will refer to them as lean tools and your EXERBAG.

CHAPTER 24
Lean Tools

YOU MAY FEEL overwhelmed with all the information, processes, and recommendations thus far. Don't worry. This is normal. After engaging in the prep, the steps, and the processes, in time, you will see results and become comfortable with the whole deal. Eventually, you will become an expert on you.

To become an expert on you, there are tools to use along the journey that will help you get to know yourself and win the battle against obesity.

Getting to know yourself refers to having knowledge about your body and its responses to exercise, food, restriction, supplementation, and rest. Knowledge is power. Power to keep the momentum train moving forward. To tackle the next hurdle, and the next, and the next. Knowledge is learned through trial and error, practicing, training, reading, observing, following, measuring, monitoring, recording, and experimenting with everything involved in your weight loss journey. Knowledge and experience lead to becoming skilled. Skilled in controlling your body composition, fuel, work, play, and sleep. When you have done this for a few months, you start to notice trends, changes, and responses in your body that you can self-control through macronutrient manipulation, exercise timing, thoughts and behavior, supplementation, fasted cardio, and weightlifting.

Getting to know your body and learning how to control its physical attributes is something we should work on when we are young, but it is not a subject taught in school. At least not to the extent this book delivers.

Another way to put it is that you need to monitor you . . . clinically monitor you. This requires tools and devices to capture data like your weight and blood pressure, then journaling to record all your data, feelings, and results. This process of data collection, observation, and recording what is happening to your body when you exercise and eat can let you review it to gain knowledge on what works and what doesn't, what worked really well, and what to keep doing or never do again.

In a hospital, there are certain numbers that matter the most when it comes to your body. Your doctor can externally control or influence these numbers nurses collect and monitor through IV fluids, pharmaceuticals, food, activity, or bed rest. Yup, your medical team can actually physically change your body weight, heart rate, blood sugar, blood pressure, lipid levels, sodium, and potassium, to shit or not to shit, and rather fast. *Holy hell*, you might be saying to yourself, *this is frickin' crazy*. No. It's human physiology, science, and chemistry. This is exactly why you too can monitor and control some of these physiological parameters at home through over-the-counter means, nutrition control, macronutrient manipulation, and body monitoring tools. Maximize self-awareness. You do not need your doctor to tell you what your blood pressure or heart rate is. The same goes for blood sugar, blood oxygen, ketosis monitoring, or your ability to take pooping aids. The tools to check these vitals and blood chemistry are widely available and affordable nowadays, and there is no excuse to *not* take responsibility for yourself and your health. Every person should monitor these basics at home and when there is a problem, contact their doctor.

Wipe your own! Right?

Self-monitoring leads to self-regulation and habit and behavior change. Self-monitoring is key to the process and brings deliberate attention to the main aspects of how dieting and exercise affect you. By observing with your own eyes, feeling with your own hands, and collecting data, you can correlate positive changes with actual personal behavior and actions, which leads to affirmation in your power over self. Self-regulation depends on you being honest. Do not lie to yourself when recording data. Self-monitoring also must be regular, routine, and timely. This process will lead to personal performance measures you can count on. You can control you, your weight, your strength, and your wellness (National Institutes of Health/NIH. www.ncbi.nlm.nih.gov).

You can go all out and monitor everything under the sun or limit your data collection and monitoring to the minimum necessary.

Let's go over some things you should monitor during your war against obesity and the equipment or tools you'll need to do so.

1. Body weight: scale
2. Naked observation: mirror; journal with pictures in swimsuit
3. Blood pressure: home blood pressure unit
4. Heart rate and blood oxygen: finger pulse oximeter
5. Steps: fitness watch (Fitbit, GPS watch, or other smart watch)
6. Ketones: ketosis test strips
7. BMI, BMR, body fat, waist-to-hip ratio, ideal weight, TDEE, THR (target heart rate), 1RM (rep max): calculator applications and formulas
8. Waist, neck, thigh, buttocks, calf, biceps, and chest circumference measurements: tape measure
9. Body fat thickness: body caliper
10. Quick body fat percentage tester: bioelectrical impedance analysis
11. Blood sugar: glucose monitoring device (for diabetics)
12. Feelings, thoughts, pain, fatigue, and subjective perspectives, good and bad: journal

Let's go over the tools of the trade and the benefits you will attain by using them in your program.

The Scale

If you don't monitor your weight when executing the EXERLEAN formula, you will burn off body fat and lose body weight regardless. You can use feeling and observation like watching how loose your clothing is getting, and the benefits will be obvious. So if this is the case, then why weigh yourself?

Body weight can be a controversial topic, so some say that monitoring weight is unnecessary and should be avoided. This is ludicrous! If you lost 5 pounds, wouldn't you like to know it? There is no benefit to purposefully being *unaware* of your body weight. There are costs, though, like the inability to calculate BMI, lean body mass, body fat percentage, BMR/RMR, and TDEE and then continue to monitor changes and adjust the variables as necessary to maximize outcomes.

If you cannot calculate your BMR or lean body mass, you cannot plan out your calories based on real data, only guessing. If you gain lean body mass over time, then you need to increase your calorie intake to maintain it.

Checking your weight daily also allows you to see real results, even if you can't notice a difference in the mirror. It is nearly impossible for an obese person to see a difference in the mirror in the first month of dieting. Regardless, huge changes are likely occurring. Real data is always that—real and objective. You may not notice weight loss, but if you have gone from 280 to 250 pounds, that is a loss you can see with your own eyes. You can then make decisions based on the objective facts. If your scale says you went from 280 to 250, then keep doing what you are doing regardless of whether you see a difference in the mirror.

For a beginner or nonprofessional dieter, which is most people, it is crucial to monitor your body weight during a weight loss endeavor, especially in the beginning. You need to know if you're taking in the right number of calories to stoke the metabolic fire. If you are not losing weight, you are likely overconsuming and need to decrease your calories. If you are losing weight too fast, you may need to increase your daily calorie intake.

The best scales are digital and easy to use. The new smart scales not only measure your body weight but in addition calculate your BMI, lean body mass, and body fat percentage based on bioelectrical impedance, in which an electrical current travels through your fat tissue slower than it does through lean body parts. The data is displayed with charts and graphs. Because smart scales use Wi-Fi, you can link one with your smart watch to also incorporate step count, heart rate, and sleep data. This is the route I take and recommend. I use the Fitbit Ionic, the Fitbit Aria 2 Wi-Fi Smart Scale, and a handheld Omron bioelectrical impedance monitor. If you're considering a bioelectrical impedance monitor and have an electrical implant like a pacemaker, or if you are pregnant, consult your doctor first.

The Mirror

The mirror is also an excellent tool to monitor truth. What you look like naked in the mirror is the real deal. This cannot be manipulated, adjusted, cropped, refinished, or edited. The mirror does not lie. You may be able to minimize obesity with cosmetics and clothing, but the truth will always remain underneath. When you lose body fat, you will notice changes in the way you look naked and the way your clothing fits. People around you will start to notice, too: "Are you losing weight?"

I can tell you firsthand that the mirror is my most beneficial tool because through the process of cutting, I can observe with my own eyes the truth. There is nothing more rewarding than seeing your body physically change for the better as a result of remaining disciplined in eating restrictively, exercising, and finishing the prep work. "You did this," you can say to yourself. The mirror validates the process, your effort, and your sacrifices.

As you get older, you may need two mirrors, one in front and one behind, working in sync to do exactly that . . . see your behind! It is important to have a good-quality, full-length mirror to avoid distortions or bent images and to see your full body accurately from head to toe.

The selfie of a mirror reflection is popular nowadays, especially after you just killed it in the gym. You can position yourself in the best way with just the right light, then snap that selfie. This is a good way to monitor your progress. Another way to monitor your progress is to take a picture of yourself in underwear, in skimpy clothing, or hell, naked—the truest image of yourself.

Whatever format you choose, you should take a whole-body selfie daily to monitor progress. Three months from your start date, you can look back on your pictures. If you remain true to the EXERLEAN program and make the necessary sacrifices, then you will see an amazing transformation underway. This proof of concept will in turn fuel your motivation train to help get you through another three months, then another three months, and so on.

Costco, Walmart, Target, and other department stores sell good full-length mirrors. If you have a handyperson around or are handy yourself, you can purchase a large raw mirror from Home Depot or Lowe's and mount it to your wall with construction adhesive and mirror clips. This method is my preference as I was able to set up a small wall of mirrors in my home gym for great self-portraits . . . and flexing.

Home Blood Pressure Unit

Every adult on this earth should monitor their blood pressure regularly. The older you get, the more often you should take your blood pressure. When you are beginning an exercise, weightlifting, and dieting regimen, you should monitor your blood pressure daily for the first month so you have a present awareness of how your body is physiologically responding.

According to the American Heart Association, normal blood pressure is 120/80, elevated is higher than this, and hypertension is considered 130/80 or higher. Low blood pressure is defined as 90/60 or lower (mayoclinic.org) If you have abnormally high blood pressure, typically over 130/80, you should consult your primary care doctor because you may have a heart or body chemistry problem that needs attending to. Same goes for low blood pressure or if either high or low blood pressure is accompanied by lightheadedness or dizziness. High blood pressure can lead to brain bleeds, heart attacks, and other health problems. Low blood pressure can lead to passing out, low oxygen to vital organs including the brain, and poor circulation. Consult your doctor if you feel off. Prevention is key when dealing with blood pressure.

Home blood pressure units are available online and in most pharmacies, department stores, and other retailers. They are affordable and easy to use in the comfort of your own home, all automated with no doctor or nurse needed.

Pulse Oximeter

This small electronic device is placed over your fingertip and will display your present heart rate and blood oxygen level. You can use the data from an oximeter to monitor what your heart is doing before, during, and after exercise. This can help you adjust your activity level, intensity, or difficulty to maintain your target heart rate.

The main attribute of the oximeter that is useful for you is the oxygen sensor. This sensor gives another readout for the oxygen saturation in your blood—basically, what percentage of oxygen is in your blood. One hundred percent oxygen in the blood indicates perfect health. Less than 100 percent is lack of oxygen in the blood. After nineteen years of working in cardiopulmonary rehab, I can tell you that 100 percent oxygen is rare.

The average person in good health seems to run 97–99 percent blood oxygen. When things start going south, blood oxygen dips below 90 percent. When a person's blood oxygen dips below 90 percent, they are in a state of hypoxia, meaning they lack enough oxygen to feed all the body's vital organs. Especially important is the brain. Hypoxia in the long run can lead to death of brain cells, dementia, cognitive impairment, and other body ailments.

For example, if you have a lung disease like cystic fibrosis, asthma, chronic obstructive pulmonary disease (COPD), or emphysema as well as congestive heart failure (CHF) or sleep apnea, you may be dipping below 90 percent blood oxygen whenever you are engaging in exertional work or exercise like weeding, shoveling snow, chopping firewood, or running on a treadmill. You don't know that you are or are not hypoxic unless you monitor yourself. People with diminished lung capacity may intermittently be in a hypoxic state and unaware of it for years. This starves the brain of necessary oxygen concentrations and over time can lead to dementia, cognitive impairment, and other diseases.

Now add in a weight training, exercise, and dieting regime. The last thing you want to be is below 90 percent when you are engaging in deadlifts or fasted cardio. If you have COPD, CHF, asthma, or another respiratory disease or problem, you should consult your doctor regularly, especially before you initiate your exercise and dieting program.

The oximeter is a simple, affordable, and easy-to-use device that you can use to monitor your body and increase self-awareness of how it is responding to diet, exercise, work, and ADL and IADL. The benefits of using an oximeter far outweigh the cost of the device.

An oximeter is available at most large pharmacies, Costco, Walmart, Amazon, and other retailers. The cheaper models may not be as accurate, but they are accurate enough for the purposes of your body transformation and body awareness.

Fitness Watch

There are many brands of fitness watches, and each has its own set of high-tech functions and data collection for tracking fitness and health. Like an oximeter, the benefits of wearing a fitness watch far outweigh the cost of purchasing one. The fitness watch has GPS function and links to your cell phone, Wi-Fi, Bluetooth, and satellites to monitor your distance and elevation changes. Some watches will add topographical mapping, path tracking, speed, and other nifty data.

Fitness watches give you an LED readout for your step count, distance traveled, weather reports, calories burned, quality of sleep, calorie consumption, and body vitals like your current heart rate and average heart rate, body temperature, and other cardiac monitoring. Not all fitness watches have all available functions, but most have the basic necessities for your transformation program, and some of the more expensive ones track everything under the sun. Of course, the watch that has the most data on you is going to be the best, but the best is not necessary for the EXERLEAN program. Your fitness watch should monitor heart rate, sleep, steps, and other GPS data. Everything else is a bonus.

A fitness watch can be purchased at most retailers and online. You should check with your employer on this one as many employers offer fitness watches as a benefit in their employee health and wellness plans.

Ketosis Test Strips

As you know, during any restrictive diet or fat-burning plan that involves eliminating carbohydrates, it is essential to monitor ketosis. As we talked about in the chapter on achieving the State of ultimate body fat incineration, we need to reach a state of ketosis, then hover just out of it. The most accurate method of identifying ketosis is with ketosis test strips.

Testing for ketosis is accomplished by dipping the ketosis test strip in your urine stream once or twice a day during carbohydrate restriction. You can be confident in your carbohydrate restriction while monitoring with ketosis test strips. When your body starts spilling ketones into your urine, then you know you're in or entering ketosis and can make the necessary changes to get out of it and then hover there. This is the State.

Calculator Applications

Pre-, during, and post-EXERLEAN, then every so often for the rest of your life during a maintenance phase, you should monitor and track these important statistics:

- BMI
- BMR

- Body fat percentage
- Waist-to-hip ratio
- Ideal weight
- TDEE
- THR
- 1RM

Before the start date of your program, you should have gathered all these body composition stats and appearance data. It is too late to get your preprogram pictures after you have executed your exercise and diet. You will lose a larger percentage of body weight and body fat at the start of a diet and exercise regimen, so you want to make sure you record all these data markers. They will be your baseline and the reference point for all future measurements and calculations.

The calculators for many of these can be found online, some in apps, and in the future on the front page of www.exerlean.com. Remember to write down all your beginning data in your program journal and then have a backup of the data and pictures in case you misplace them or if something unforeseen happens, like the dog ate them.

Tape Measure

A tape measure is a cheap tool for gathering valuable body dimension data. It is vital to measure all your main limb and trunk circumferences and record the data to establish your baseline body volume metrics. Make sure you purchase one long enough to wrap the entirety of your abdomen, buttocks, and chest.

When measuring your body parts, record with your body part in the relaxed and fullest position. Do not squeeze or tighten the tape measure to make the measurement smaller than it really is; the measurement must be an accurate recording of the body part. Record the dimension or circumference of the biggest area of girth, muscle belly, or fat, which should be the center of the muscle belly unless you are oddly shaped or super-morbidly obese. If you take measurements from an off-center area, write this down, and if possible, have someone take a picture of you measuring yourself. By doing this, you can know that you are always measuring the same spot every time you periodically monitor progress throughout your fat-burning journey.

Here is a list of the areas of your body you need to measure and record:

1. **Left and right calves.** Measure the biggest portion of your calf, flexed and relaxed.
2. **Left and right thighs.** Measure the biggest area/largest circumference, flexed and relaxed.
3. **Hip-to-hip width and circumference.** Measure at the iliac crest (the largest part of your hip/pelvic bone).
4. **Waistline/belly circumference.** Measure at the naval and if you have a larger section than that, take additional detailed records and pictures of that location too.
5. **Chest.** Wrap the tape measure around your back and under your armpits to the front of your chest. Measure the center of the pectoralis (pecs) muscle belly, flexed and relaxed. Women should also measure the biggest area of breast circumference.
6. **Back.** Wrap the tape measure around your back and under your armpits to the front of your chest. This time pull the tape measure into the uppermost area in the armpits and upper latissimus (lats). Measure your lats flared out/flexed and relaxed.
7. **Left and right forearms.** Measure the largest area, or muscle belly, of your forearm.
8. **Left and right upper arms or biceps/triceps.** Measure at largest area in the center of your biceps and around your triceps. Make sure the tape is not angled or diagonal but straight across and around from biceps to triceps. Record your arm flexed and relaxed.
9. **Neck.** (Measure around the largest area center of neck)
10. **Head.** Take two measurements: one under your chin or jawbone and over the top of your head, then back down to your chin (essentially your face shape), and the second from just above your eyebrows over your ears to the back of your head, like you would for your hat size.
11. **Other.** If you have any other body part you want to monitor for change during the program, like fat feet, make a detailed record and take pictures to ensure you're measuring the same area every time. You have only one chance to gather as much preprogram data as you can. You'll never be this bad off again, so take advantage of all the ways you can record yourself through pictures, measurements, and

all the other lean tools available. You're about to witness epic changes. Future you is on the horizon!

It may seem odd to measure some of these areas, but trust me, your head measurements as well as all other measurements will shrink as you burn off body fat. Most people are clueless as to the actual amount of fat on their bodies, including odd areas like your face, head, armpits, low back, groin, and feet. It is amazing how much better you look and feel when these areas are lean.

Tape measure data and pictures tell the truth. Down the road, when you're doing a physical self-checkup and collecting data, it will be very rewarding when you see the numbers shrinking. Oh hell, yeah . . . shrinking! Doesn't that sound good?

Body Caliper

This tool measures skin-fold thickness to calculate body fat. You enter your caliper measurements into an online calculator or use the formulas available with the product and manually calculate body fat percentage yourself. You can find a caliper method calculator at https://exrx.net/Calculators/BodyComp and www.linear-software.com/online.html.

The body caliper is the most accurate method of calculating body fat percentage since it basically "pinches" your skin. There are different methods to complete the test, each using a different amount of skin-fold measurements in various locations on your body. The one with the most skin-fold measures of nine different pinch sites is the most accurate. Sometimes it is not possible to record some areas of the body if you are too fat. If this is the case, then the tape measure, bioimpedance, BMI calculator, and pictures will suffice.

Gym-quality or healthcare-quality calipers are cost prohibitive, but you can get a cheap plastic set online that will work just fine. It will usually come with a chart and instructions for how to complete the test. Add pic of body calipers here.

Bioelectric Impedance Analysis

Bioelectrical impedance body fat analysis sends an electric current through your body to sense the proportions of lean mass versus body fat based on your body's resistance to the electric current. Bioelectrical impedance analysis (BIA) is not the most accurate method of body composition analysis, but it works. I have found that it tends to score high when compared to the body caliper analysis. Some research demonstrates that BIA reads low or high depending on when your last meal was eaten or if you exercised beforehand.

Regardless, the good thing about using bioelectrical impedance to monitor body fat status is that it is a quick, easy method and will show a change up or down if you gained or lost body fat, respectively. As long as your body weight and body fat percentage are trending downward, you can pat yourself on the back and continue doing what you are doing because it is working. And vice versa—if you are dieting to lose weight, and a couple weeks have passed and the numbers are not changing, then you can decrease calories, carbs, and/or fat intake until you start burning off body fat and losing weight. If the numbers or measurements from the bioelectrical impedance device are going up, you are getting fatter. If the numbers are going down, you are getting leaner. If they are not moving, neither is your body fat.

There are many BIA devices available online and in retail stores. I have used an Omron handheld device and currently use the Fitbit Aria 2. Both devices do the job. I recommend you research the customer reviews on whatever BIA devices interest you, and go with the one that has great customer satisfaction.

Glucose Monitoring Device

If you have diabetes, blood sugar monitoring is the most important thing you can do to make sure your blood glucose levels remain within normal range. Diabetics are at high risk of heart attacks, strokes, kidney disease, blindness, circulation problems, wounds, ulcers, and body part amputation.

The American Diabetes Association (ADA) target blood sugar levels are 80–130 mg/dl premeal and below 180 mg/dl one to two hours after a meal. The ADA also recommends working with your doctor to identify your personal blood sugar goals based on your individual status and circumstances.

Nondiabetics can also benefit from monitoring their blood sugar levels, for example, to test for hyperglycemia, insulin resistance, or prediabetic conditions. Blood sugar monitoring is not necessary for nondiabetics, but at minimum, you should get a yearly health review by your primary care doctor to make sure your body is functioning properly.

You can test yourself at home using an electronic device called a glucose meter or glucometer. The glucometer can test your blood sugar levels before, during, and after exercise and meals and before and after sleep. This will give you a better understanding of how your body responds to exercise, dieting, and sleep. The more aware of your body you are, the better able you will be to control your body composition, energy levels, sleep, and performance through nutrition and exercise.

If you do use a glucometer, I recommend you record all the data and timing of data, whether it was before or after a meal, exercise, or sleep. Then take this information to your next doctor appointment for review. If your numbers fall outside the ADA's recommendations, seek advice and counseling from your doctor as soon as possible.

Journal

Keeping a detailed journal is one of the most important tools during your healthstyle transformation and weight loss journey. Journaling is important in goal setting and achievement for business, work, lifestyle transformation, dieting, exercise, sports, and many other realms of human advancement. Writing down your thoughts, feelings, daily events, weight, strength gains, diet, exercise, failures, and mistakes, reviewing your goals, and recording anything else you feel the need to will help you maintain a state of mindfulness, focus, think productively, and remain organized for the mission at hand. Journaling is a record of events and important data, an assembly of the highlights in your life to use for recollection as you plan your next move.

For your EXERLEAN transformation, you should journal daily even if it's just a quick summary of the day's events. So, what to write down?

1. **Thoughts and feelings.** It is important to follow how you feel because you can acknowledge trends in your diet, exercise, and sleep that may need adjustment to steer your mind out of the dark and into the light. We need to listen to our bodies, and to do this, we must decipher the messages our thoughts and feelings represent. Low blood sugar,

vitamin deficiencies, excessive calorie restriction, ghrelin's a yellin', lack of sleep, and overconsumption are all good examples of a push of inspiration from our body. Call it intuition, body awareness, introspection, or mind-body connection—the process is real.

2. **Daily calories.** You must keep track of your daily calorie intake so you can connect the dots between weight gain, weight loss, and your calories per hour (CPH) or daily consumption. This is a summary of your protein, carbohydrate, and fat intake.

3. **Daily carbs.** Carbohydrate intake is the main variable you need to monitor and adjust to achieve the State of ultimate body fat incineration. An accurate carb count along with grams of fat and protein will allow you to keep track of your daily calorie intake. How many grams a day? What is the glycemic rating? The timing of carbs specifically for your last meal, making sure that you are not consuming carbs too close to sleep?

4. **Daily fat.** EXERLEAN's goal is low fat intake, so keep track of grams of fat a day, including healthy fat supplementation.

5. **Protein intake.** It is important to consume enough protein to maintain a positive nitrogen state. How many grams of protein a day? What is the biological value of the protein?

6. **Ketosis monitoring.** Until you figure out how your body performs on a low-carb diet, it is vital to monitor for ketosis. Record the level of ketosis and at what day, hour, or point you finally entered ketosis. How many low-GI carbs did it take to get out of ketosis? What ratio of carbs is necessary to hover just out of ketosis but not to the point of glycogen replenishment? I recommend starting by adding 25 grams of low-glycemic carbs for two meals and see if that gets you out of ketosis. Fifty grams, or 200 calories (4 calories per gram) derived from low-GI carbs, is a good start to see where you need to be. Depending on your BMR, you may need more or less, but that remains to be determined through weeks of trial and error. If you are spilling ketones when you test your urine the next day, add another 25 grams to a third meal. If not, stick with 50 grams. As long as you're losing weight and not in ketosis, you're likely right where you need to be. If you are small framed or short, 50 grams a day may be too much, and you will need to decrease your carbs until you start spilling ketones again, then add a few more until you are out of

ketosis on a daily basis. This process of trial and error will continue until you get a clear picture of your body function, your metabolic set points, and your fat-burning zone.
7. **Daily cardio.** What exercise? What machine? How many minutes? What level of resistance? Incline level? Speed? You will appreciate this data down the road when you are in much better condition and can see that it has paid off.
8. **Weightlifting.** What body parts on what day? How many repetitions? How many sets? What was your max weight you resisted? With the EXERLEAN Weight Chaining protocol, you will get stronger. You will improve your lean muscle build and tone. You will improve your metabolism. You will harness greater energy and endurance. These benefits are all worth noting in your journal.
9. **Sleep.** If you have a smart watch or Fitbit that monitors your sleep pattern, you might find it beneficial to keep track of the different stages of sleep. How much REM, rested, and awake hours you were during your sleep. You may be able to look at all the nutrition data in your journal and in time figure out what nutrition profile promotes your best sleep quality.
10. **Body weight.** This real number demonstrates whether what you are doing is working or not working. Always record your weight at the same time every day. I recommend recording it twice a day, first thing in the morning on an empty stomach before any activity after you urinate, then directly before bed after urinating. All other times of the day will fluctuate greatly due to water, sodium, and nutritional intake.
11. **Bioelectrical impedance.** This should be done at the same time every day. I recommend recording your body fat percentage first thing in the morning on an empty stomach.
12. **Body fat calipers.** Record once a week or every two weeks.
13. **Tape measurements.** Measure your main body parts once a month. When you see that you are shrinking, you will know your hard work and sacrifice are paying off.
14. **Weekly pictures.** Take as many before pictures and videos of yourself as you can. In addition to your program's beginning, middle, and end pictures and videos, add three weekly pics to your journal—front, back, and side profiles. Try to wear the same outfit from beginning

to end, whether your program is three months or three years, to see your progress over time.

You should add anything in your journal that you feel may help you on your quest to becoming master and commander of your physical body and life choices. Journaling is a long-used tool by some of the most celebrated and influential people who have walked the earth. As an example, the Bible is a journal of events detailing humanity's encounters with God, the plans and commandments delivered, and the sacrifice then resurrection of the messiah Jesus Christ. The Bible is the number one selling book in the history of mankind—all from years of journaling combined into a book. Trust me on this one, your journal, your book, will be influential for you and others when you do the work and prove that it is possible to conquer resistance and change yourself enigmatically.

CHAPTER 25
EXERBAG: Your Gym Bag Essentials

Any gym, whether on a beach, in a home, or in a commercial building, is a place that has exercise equipment arranged in a way to streamline your workout. No matter the gym, you will find yourself unprepared without the basic gym essentials. The gym essentials are the items that make your workout safer and comfortable and that facilitate the exercise process. Nobody wants to be that person who shows up to the gym empty-handed.

To truly be successful in executing a monumental workout session, you should have these basic gym essentials, which are usually carried in a designated gym bag. For EXERLEAN, that's your EXERBAG. Here is what to consider for your gym bag and some of the basic items in a seasoned weightlifter's EXERBAG.

1. **Gym bag.** You need a good bag to carry and protect your clothing, wallet or purse, epic workout gear, and whatever else you bring. Don't use a low-quality bag that will fall apart. You're in this for the long haul and need a lasting product. Be sure to choose one that will fit all your gear. I have found great deals on high-quality gear at Big 5 Sporting Goods, Walmart, and online at www.amazon.com (search "bodybuilding gym bags").

2. **Workout gloves.** For one, a good set of workout gloves provide a barrier to protect your hands. They will help prevent ripping the skin, spreading germs, and acquiring tough callouses. Workout gloves also improve your grip on the bar, dumbbells, kettlebells, machines, balls, bags, and ropes. Workout gloves come in many different styles, colors, materials, and levels of sturdiness. Some have aeration to allow skin to breathe, gel padding for comfort, and gripping material

stitched into the palm side. Some gloves even have lifting straps or hooks built into them just in case you need to lift or push some crazy heavy weights. I prefer wristwrap gloves, which have an extra-long strap that wraps around your wrist to give it greater stability during weightlifting. Whatever gloves you decide to put in your EXERBAG, you will appreciate having them when it is workout time. I use the Harbinger Pro WristWrap Gloves.

3. **Water bottle.** It is important to drink water during your workout . . . a lot of water! Water hydrates your muscles, lubricates your joints, and is a necessary component in the metabolic pathway. Instead of making a hundred trips to the water bubbler, keep your water bottle right there with you. Any water bottle will suffice, but I have found the best bottle is one that will fit in the cupholder on any machine. I sometimes bring a larger one on a grinding bodybuilding day.

4. **Weightlifting belt.** Protect your belly. Protect your spine. That's why the weightlifting belt is the most valuable item in your gym bag. The weightlifting belt wraps around your upper waist and lumbar spine area to help keep everything together. Unless you are already in great shape, with tight abdominals and a strong core, you are at high risk of sustaining an abdominal or supraumbilical hernia (under your belly button), straining, or injuring your spine.

Weightlifting belts come in many shapes and sizes. I recommend wearing as wide and as thick of a belt that's still comfortable. The gold standard is a four-inch belt. What works best for you just depends on your body shape, strength, and level of intensity. If you are too big to wear one, that is okay—you are working toward being able to wear one. Just remember to always keep proper form to help prevent injury until you purchase one.

Weightlifting belts can get costly. You don't need an expensive belt, though. You just need a good weightlifting belt that works. I have invested in a few to use during different styles of lifting. I use a light-duty fabric and easy-to-adjust belt with a Velcro strap for lighter-weight and quicker-moving lifts. I have a four-inch backup medium-duty fabric belt from Rogue Fitness to use if I feel like it. My go-to belt is my heavy-duty four-inch Cardillo bodybuilding/power-lifting belt for deadlifts, squats, and most everything else.

5. **Workout-specific shoes.** Weightlifting or exercising in thick, squishy, tall-soled running shoes is a no-no. And no high heels in the gym! No open-toe shoes! No slippers! No aqua shoes! Say hello to a twisted or rolled ankle, broken toes, or other injury.

    Running or tennis shoes are good for cardio machines, calisthenics, running, and select weightlifting that does not involve the legs. Running shoes are lighter and feel best when on the elliptical trainer, treadmill, stair mill, or ripping through a body weight workout.

    For weightlifting or powerlifting, you want designated shoes. Weightlifting shoes are usually midtop or high-top to support the ankle better. The sole is the opposite of a running shoe. It is firm and thinner, and it bites into the floor during a heavy lift. Your feet will greatly appreciate a good set of cardio shoes and a separate set of shoes built for weight training. If you cannot afford both, I recommend getting the weightlifting shoes or high-tops with ankle support, like a good set of Otomix weightlifting shoes, Under Armour's Project Rock Delta, or other basketball-style or football-style high-tops with a sturdy sole. If you can afford both, then go for it . . . you're worth the investment.

    Running shoes are more finicky and should be tried on and walked in before purchasing. I have found great benefit from the Hoka One One shoes for work since I'm walking on concrete floors all day and also for cardiovascular exercise at the gym. But I repeat, I would not wear these for weightlifting that involves my legs for support.

6. **Exercise- and bodybuilding-friendly clothing.** Don't wear jeans to the gym. It's just wrong. In reality, though, it doesn't matter what you wear to the gym as long as you are there and killing the weights. But please, consider taking the time to dress in something that will help you endure the session. If you are uncomfortable when exercising or weightlifting, you won't last very long in the gym. Wear clothing that is lightweight, comfortable, breathable, and supportive of the activity. What you find comfortable to wear during a workout is totally personal. I love going to a gym and seeing all the different styles and preferences. It's a great demonstration of the eclectic blend of fashions and personas. I prefer to wear workout pants and a thin,

well-fitting T-shirt for weight training, then shorts if I'm hitting cardio. Pants provide extra skin protection, especially on a deadlift day.

7. **Music and headphones.** Music reaches the subconscious mind. It motivates, boosts thought intensity, and helps us surpass our perceived endurance limit. Lifting weights to powerful music or hearing our favorite tunes while engaging in a bout of cardio helps make that time more enjoyable. Also, time will pass much quicker than it will from hearing other people and gym equipment banging about. Podcasts and audiobooks are also great for cardio. Aside from the obvious positive benefits of music for personal pleasure and workout motivation, wearing headphones or earbuds—even if the music is off—deters others from asking you questions or striking up a conversation. These distractions will just prolong your workout, pull you off track, and diminish the quality of your work. Distracted workout sessions lead to a loss of intensity and focus. The gym is not social hour . . . get shit done, then visit, then leave. You've got other more productive things to do after this. Speaking of productivity, if you use your phone instead of an MP3 player to listen to music, be sure not to use it for anything else, like checking social media.

8. **Combination lock.** Have a good lock that will attach to whatever lockers are offered at the gym you decide to enroll in. Don't leave your gym bag by the wall, in a cubby, or next to your machine. Most gyms have lockers available, first come, first served. If you are addicted to looking at social media, then put that not-so-smartphone in the locker too. There will be a huge difference in the results between 365 days of intense and focused workouts compared to 365 days of distracted workouts focused on selfies that say, "Look at me! I'm at the gym!" What will inspire people is seeing you grueling through a heavy rep, sweating beads, veins poppin', and muscles striating. That is the pic of the day.

There you go. Your EXERBAG! When you carry this baby around, you'll feel equipped and ready to tackle any gym warfare.

CHAPTER 26
Phase One: Cutting

THIS WIDESPREAD CONUNDRUM of excess fat on our bodies, imprisoning us from movement freedom and endless energy, must end. The end comes with executing a cutting phase of massive proportion.

Bodybuilders go through phases of body composition through their competition life cycle. The first phase is a bulking or mass-building phase, where the goal is to add lean muscle mass through grueling weight-lifting repetitions and massive high BV protein and low-GI carbohydrate consumption. The second phase is a maintenance phase, where the bodybuilder gives maximum effort in the gym and leans out the diet of excess fat and carbs yet maintains high protein volume until they initiate the third phase, cutting.

The cutting phase carves away all the fat on the body through thermogenesis—the State. The bodybuilder does this to take off the "fat suit" then showcase their newly earned muscle-bound physique in the next bodybuilding competition. There is no better knowledge on fat burning than that of a seasoned competitive bodybuilder, with their unseen secret strategies and processes.

No matter what phase of body composition you are seeking, you are a bodybuilder too. You and me . . . bodybuilders. We are all bodybuilders. Some of us compete on the stage, some of us don't. Regardless, we all showcase our physiques publicly throughout life. Do you want to showcase an obese body, or do you want to strut your stuff in a lean, healthy physique?

If you do the work to gain body fat and become obese, then you built your body that way . . . didn't you?

If you eat lean, lift heavy weights, and eat a lot of protein, then you are building something . . . right?

Being a bodybuilder doesn't necessarily mean you have to slip into a banana hammock and get on stage and strike an archer pose. No. We are all bodybuilders minus the banana hammock or sparkly G-string bikini. It's just that we are all building different body types. Some of us sacrifice and engineer our bodies into the best state of health and athleticism we can. Some of us don't give a shit; instead, we have given up and given in to resistance, the highly addictive state of sedentary behavior, and hyper-palatable food overconsumption.

Who are you?

What body are you building?

What body are you going to build next?

This book is designed to help with one thing and one thing only. To change your health and wellness for life. Transformation.

This first step in this operation is to treat obesity. To change the way you live, adopt a new healthstyle for life, and do the work necessary to earn your lean, healthy body. Cutting body fat at all costs is the mission. No turning back. No cheating. No fatback.

The EXERLEAN protocol for fat burning, the State, may not only help cure your obesity but also help you gain new muscle mass, increase your resting metabolic rate, and improve your libido and your stamina for ADL, IADL, and work. If you do the work, execute the EXERLEAN protocol, maintain focus and discipline, eat clean, and persevere, you will win.

Don't count yourself out. Don't give up. If not now, you may someday realize that you too are a bodybuilder. Can you imagine getting lean and in the best shape of your life? You may just want to showcase that shit in a competition someday. It happens; modifying your body for the better is addictive. I've had many friends, clients, and family members get ripped through strategic cutting, then jump on the stage in a bodybuilding show.

Your successful transformation will inspire others. Weight loss is rare these days and highly motivating for others because your success becomes proof of concept. Change your body in epic proportions, then get ready for the onslaught of attention and self-help questions from those inspired by your success story.

This is what I want for you. I want you to feel the monumental positivity that comes with earning a lean body through restriction, discipline, and hard work. Easy is not motivating for anyone, and any diet program that seems *easy* is bullshit and a waste of time. All those diets on the covers of magazines, on blogs, and on social media that promote easy and massive weight loss in a short amount of time are all propaganda and deception. Don't fall for this ruse. The work . . . the restriction . . . the suffering . . . the sacrifice must be endured to achieve real results.

You know this. We all know this. But still, we are attracted to the least restrictive path, the easy road, the marketing. That is why most of us are overweight, obese, and morbidly obese. We have stopped working. Our culture has blossomed into an obese state, the Obesiboomers. This has happened because storing fat is easy to do and a bitch to get rid of. Because once it's sitting on our asses, it doesn't want to leave. We are succumbing to Alexa, power windows, power doors, escalators, elevators, hoverboards, power wheelchairs, and scooters. We are overconsuming fake food, sugary drinks, alcohol, weed, cigarettes, and fat-laden, hyper-palatable, calorie-dense processed foods. No wonder we are fat, right?

If you are overweight or obese, cutting is the only phase you should execute. When all your fat has been treated, then maintenance of your new lean and healthy body is the next and final step in your successful healthstyle transformation. Whether it takes months or years to finally achieve your healthy BMI, body fat percentage, BMR, strength, and endurance, it is vital you stick with the entire process. Beginning to end, you must overcome resistance, subdue addiction, and end victorious.

So don't worry about a bulk phase or maintenance phase at this point. Unless you yearn for bodybuilding competition or have an unrealized ambition to gain maximal muscle mass and strength, then bulking will never enter your healthstyle plan. When you have met your body transformation goal, maintenance is key to hold on to your gains, your body fat loss, and your new physique status.

When you complete your mission. Which you will.

Keep what you have earned.

Maintain this epic state at all costs.

CHAPTER 27
Phase Two: Maintenance

WHEN YOU ARE walking around in a lighter, leaner, miraculous you, maintaining this phenomenon is the final stage in your journey of physical transformation. Maintenance for life, you might say. Living in a maintenance phase is the ultimate health objective. Being in a maintenance phase means you have a lean, healthy physique and are committed to the work necessary to live at your best—daily, weekly, monthly, yearly, decadal, until death. You are maintaining personal fitness and vitality by staying active and laboring. You are eating lean and restrictively, creating occasional voids that can be replenished with a rare treat, off-diet food, or eating out. Do the work and earn the payout. That is maintenance.

It is much easier to maintain a lean, healthy physique than it is to attain it when you're obese or out of shape. Lose the body fat, then keep it off. This is the goal.

So, how do you maintain after you lose all the weight?

The answer is simple: don't change anything too much. If what you have been doing delivered you to a beautiful place, why deviate?

If maintenance is on your mind, you have likely endured months to years of work and have finally met your body weight and composition goals. Future you has become present you. If this is the case, congratulations. Fist bump and a high five. You did the work. You earned this. Welcome to the 1 percent.

Now keep it at all costs.

Maintaining a lean physique is where most fail, bouncing back in glorific obese face stuffing and other avenues of self-sabotage.

Not you.

No way!

I want you to think deep on this. Please, don't give in to the idea that all of a sudden, you can just eat anything you want and be more sedentary. This is what most people believe and act on. People constantly sacrifice, burn off the fat, and achieve the atypical lean body. Then soon after, they rebound to a weight higher than they were to begin with. This is because there is a myth that you can eat and do whatever you want if you are lean. This is a lie. Lean people don't overeat and live sedentary lifestyles. They eat lean and purposefully. They are the opposite of sedentary. They are active, not lazy. Otherwise, they would be fat.

You did the work; now keep working until you die. Fight for your health. Fight to stay lean and active. Because the day you give in or give up is the end of your glory phase. Getting fat is so frickin' easy that you should not even tempt the goddess of obesity or she will overtake you and your will to live lean. Fight like your life depends on it. Because it does.

To maintain your lean, healthy body, remain active. Keep eating lean. Keep thinking and doing things that promote a healthy lifestyle.

- Don't smoke.
- Don't overdrink alcohol.
- Don't overeat.
- Avoid desserts, candy, pastas, and breads.
- Seek protein and fibrous vegetables.
- Don't allow undeserved, unearned sedentary time.
- Go to bed early, sleep well, wake up early.
- Stay active.

You have mastered the State of body fat incineration and have come to know your body and how it works. How it responds to certain foods, weight training, and cardio. Take this knowledge and use it to your advantage.

So, what to do first?

You have met your transformation goal. You are lean, active, and healthy. You have increased your lean body mass, strength, and endurance. You are mentally clear, focused, and ready to take on another challenge.

First, understand that you don't have to change a thing. You are poised to get even leaner, stronger, and better than you imagined in the first place. Maybe your end goal was underrated. Maybe you underestimated yourself when you were fat and weak. Now is likely the perfect time to set an advanced personal goal. To lose a little more body fat, add a little more lean muscle mass. Maybe consider tackling something like a marathon, triathlon, century ride, or mile swim, hiking the Enchantments, or competing in a bodybuilding competition. Why not? Obesity is no longer a barrier. See where this road will take you. What was once unimaginable becomes a possibility at this point.

When you win, set the bar higher and work to win again. Life begins and ends. What you do in between is up to you. At some point you decided to take a stand. To change your ways and become leaner, stronger, and happier. Now is another time to take a stand. To stand in the face of societal norms and give complacency the middle finger. You are no longer like everyone else. You have broken physical and mental barriers in which most fail. You may not realize, feel, or believe that you have become atypical . . . but you have. You completed your EXERLEAN transformation and are a different being entirely. You are now in the 1 percent. You're eating lean and restrictively, and you're gifting your body with valuable protein and vegetables. You are feeding your body with weights, fasted cardio, and sleep. Yeah, you are now unique to the status quo. I hope you can see that the mere thought of relaxing, going back to old habits, and getting fatter is failure in the making.

Obesity is killing people every day. Sedentary behavior is rampant in the herd. Fat people are everywhere and losing their functional abilities. Wipe your own. Wipe it for life.

Not everybody acquires a passion for competition, marathons, or publicity. If you have decided to settle into your new body and healthstyle but lay off the strictness, the restriction, the intensity of it all, this is okay, this is good. You have earned it. You can maintain.

All the information and processes you have learned that helped you get lean will also be key tools in your mission to stay lean and healthy. Burning off body fat by using the EXERLEAN phase one protocol—cutting, or the State—is difficult. Maintaining, not burning off, is much easier. Switching from a "get lean at all costs" phase to a "stay lean at all costs" phase is EXERLEAN phase two—maintenance for life.

There are tricks to staying lean while incorporating the types of foods restricted in a fat-burning phase. The good news is you already know these tricks:

- *Fasted cardio* to capture the body in a low blood sugar and calorie-fasted state
- *High-BV protein loading* to harness the anabolic benefits of being in a positive nitrogen state
- *Fibrous vegetable loading* to harness the benefits of feeling full and sustain a low-carb state
- *Low-GI carbohydrates* to avoid sweet blood and its corresponding insulin response
- *Low fat intake* to promote incineration of body fat for energy
- *Waking early* to add more time to your productive life
- *Going to bed early* to avoid late-day snacking, cheating on a diet, and burning the candle too long to capture the benefits of getting up early
- *Weight Chaining protocol* to promote extension of the body against gravity, which is in a lifelong effort to overtake us when we're aging
- *Supplementation* with whey protein, amino acids, and vitamin and minerals to make the weight loss journey easier and ensure the basics are met
- *Carb depletion* to attain and then seize the state of glycogen exhaustion and from that moment on destroy the enemy—obesity

The more you incorporate all these tools into your healthstyle, the easier it is to stay lean and healthy.

Always refer to the laws and principles of Bodinomics and the economy of the human body. Work leads to accomplishment and simultaneously burns fuel. Fuel is necessary for work, exercise, and other physical activity. Sedentary time needs zero energy and will allow body fat to lay dormant. Continue to work at keeping your physical and mental capacities at peak performance. Fuel your body only with what is necessary to get the work done and feel great doing it. Don't overfill the tank, or it will runneth over and fill your body fat sacks.

Use the cost-benefit analysis in all choices dealing with health and wellness—food, exercise, Weight Chaining, other activity, sleep, supplementation, relationships, and work. Using CBA to make the heavy-handed beneficial choices will ensure movement toward your goal.

Seek constantly to improve and develop your healthstyle. When engaging in self-care, ADL, IADL, work, leisure, and other life events, stay hyperactive, live with intention, and do what must be done.

You must stay vigilant and dominate your enemies. The enemies are procrastination, fear of success, fear of failure, lack of self-awareness, indolent behavior, resistance, negative external influences, negative people and naysayers, overeating, smoking, alcohol, and drugs. These enemies are relentless forces working to incapacitate you.

You must win.

Your life and the quality of it relies on winning the war, slaying your enemies, and gaining full control of yourself and your actions.

The gift of free will is yours. Nobody else has this power or any power over you except God.

Let's go through a day in the life of Marco after he has accomplished his goal to get lean, adopted a renewed healthstyle, and is now maintaining in phase two.

Marco was in phase one of his EXERLEAN transformation for fourteen months. He went from a 230-pound obese, weak, and lazy person to a 170-pound leaner, stronger person living with vitality. During those fourteen months, he abolished his unhealthy obesity-reinforcing habits with habits that support fat burning and muscle building. He dominated his target heart rate during cardio.

Marco did the work.

He ignored or fired the naysayers who were constantly attempting to unsaddle him. He eliminated the negative external forces in his life, like watching TV late at night and gazing at his cell phone on to check social media. He is now surrounded with a positive environment that supports and empowers his healthstyle.

Here's Marco's schedule in phase two maintenance:

- **4:00 a.m.**—Wakes up. Thirty to forty-five minutes of fasted cardio, most days the elliptical, sometimes the treadmill or jogging. Cooks 50 grams of egg whites in a skillet with 2 cups frozen mixed veggies and 1 large cubed sweet potato fried in light olive oil. Has an Americano or drip coffee plus his vitamins for the day. Eats from 4:50 to 5:00 a.m. (Calories: 488; protein: 50 grams high BV; carbs: 38 grams low GI complex and 10 grams fibrous; fat: 4 grams omegas.)

- **5:00 a.m.**—Works on personal business, writes a book, paints, learns an instrument, dances, builds a website, makes videos, sets goals, plans, learns new skills, reads a nonfiction book, etc.
- **8:00 a.m.**—Work start time. Slams a 40-gram whey protein shake at start of work. (Calories: 165; protein: 40 grams high BV.)
- **10:30 a.m.**—Slams a 40-gram whey protein shake. (Calories: 165; protein: 40 grams high BV.)
- **12:00 p.m.**—Lunch break. 6-ounce beef steak with 2 cups stir-fry mixed veggies (fried in soy sauce) and 1 cup steamed brown rice. (Calories: 556; protein: 55 grams; carbs: 27 grams low GI and 4 grams fibrous; fat: 15 grams.)
- **4:00 p.m.**—Slams a 40-gram whey protein shake. (Calories: 165; protein: 40 grams high BV.)
- **5:00 p.m.**—Off work. Headed to the gym. Slams an NO_2 pre-workout amino acid supplement (without caffeine this late in the day). (Calories: 36; protein: 8 grams; carbs: 1.)
- **5:15 to 6:30 p.m.**—Weight Chaining workout followed by ten minutes of fasted cardio. Listens to motivational music during his workout and drowns out the external stimuli, putting all focus on attaining the prize.
- **6:30 p.m.**—Slams a 40-gram post-workout whey protein shake. (Calories: 165; protein: 40 grams high BV.)
- **7:30 p.m.**—Dinner at home. 6-ounce lean beef steak chopped up in 4 cups mixed garden fibrous vegetable salad, 1/2 avocado chopped, and 2 tablespoons light vinaigrette dressing. (Calories: 517; protein: 55 grams; carbs: 9 grams fibrous from salad, 6 grams from avocado, and 4 from vinaigrette; fat: 24 grams.)
- **9:00 p.m.**—Bedtime.

Total daily calories: 2,217

Total protein: 328 grams (secures positive nitrogen balance)

Total carbs: 94 grams (mostly low-GI carbs; Marco can add more if he needs to increase calories)

Total fat: 43 grams (intake remains low; healthy fats)

Let's look at all Marco was able to accomplish in his simple day using his new disciplined and strategic EXERLEAN healthstyle habits.

Marco completed **thirty minutes of fasted cardio** first thing in the morning. He had nearly **two hours of free time** to work on his hobbies and personal ambitions. He **worked eight full hours** at his job. He **maintained a positive nitrogen state** through high-BV protein loading. He **avoided hyperglycemia** by consuming a low to moderate amount of low-GI carbs. He **ate plenty of healthy, fibrous vegetables**. He **took his vitamins**. He **ate three full, real-food meals**. He ate no snacks and consumed no additional calories after dinner and before bed.

He **completed a Weight Chaining workout** stimulating muscle growth, strengthening, and antigravity extension. He **had one and a half hours of free time** to spend with his wife and work on his personal items in the evening before bed. This list does not include anything productive he did in between activities or during his two-to-fifteen-minute work breaks and thirty-minute lunch.

By living restricted, Marco is able to choose the heavy-handed costly choices once in a while for reward and pleasure. But not in excess. Marco has learned to maintain balance.

Marco is able to have days on occasion where he consumes more calories and can enjoy going out to eat in moderation. Days like this promote a healthy, active, and restricted healthstyle. This is the cure for obesity. This is the way to maintain a life lean and free of the negative effects obesity wreaks in our lives.

Notice how much volume Marco consumes each day. The overall calorie intake remains at a low to moderate level for an average person, but it would seem like a lot of food if you were unaware of the actual calorie amount. You wouldn't believe the number of calories an average obese person consumes a day. Over 6,000 easy. Many edging toward 10,000 at times. It's disgusting. Most obese patients I counsel are oblivious to their self-destructive indulgence and gluttony. Most are also difficult to convince otherwise.

Marco's day in the maintenance phase is focused on a high-protein positive nitrogen, low-fat, low-GI, low-carbohydrate diet, which is the easiest way to stay lean, gain more lean body tissue, and heal and rejuvenate the body.

It is not necessary, though, to engage in a high-protein diet at all times in the maintenance phase. At this point, Marco has met his goal of body transformation and just needs to maintain it. Maintenance can be done through many different nutritional strategies, including moderate to high low-GI carbs, low fat to nonfat, and moderate to high protein consumption. Try different variations of what you know works, and see what happens. You can experiment to see what macronutrient ratio works best for you. If you start getting fatter, reign in the carbs, decrease the calories, or up the protein. Do what is necessary to maintain your strong muscles and keep off body fat. You are now master controller of your body composition.

Whatever you choose, you just need to ensure any carbs are low glycemic or fibrous, all proteins are as high biological value as possible, and fat consumption is as low as possible forever. To help figure out what formula works best for you, you could consult a certified sports nutritionist, licensed nutritionist, certified health coach, or certified personal trainer at this point or design your own well-balanced diet plan based on everything you've learned in the EXERLEAN program. You've got this! Since you are lean, fit, conditioned, and healthy, maintenance will be easy, regardless of the maintenance path you decide on.

At times, Marco may need to complete a couple of weeks in the State if he notices body fat gains. At any time, you too may need to relive the EXERLEAN fat-burning algorithm to reestablish the positive effects of thermogenesis through glycogen depletion and fasting. Keep doing the two-week cycle until you reach your baseline lean state. Then maintenance again. Nobody's perfect, and we can try our best to avoid body fat, but sometimes life throws us curveballs. When this happens, it's vital to reverse the movement as soon as possible. The State will reverse obesity every time.

In the maintenance phase, you can continue to apply the principles used in the State to get lean and stay lean. Aside from your diet of abundant high BV protein, low-glycemic and fibrous carbs, and minimal fat, be sure to drink more than enough water. Engage in fasted cardio first thing in the morning on an empty stomach and weight training in the afternoon after eating all day. Keep moving, and seek active leisure adventures. Don't eat complex carbs at dinner or before bed. Go to bed early and get up early. Carb deplete or fast when necessary. Harness the power of glycogen depletion in the State if you need to incinerate some body fat.

Not everyone needs the same number of calories, carbs, protein, or fats. You will need to use all the necessary formulas and calculators to figure out your basal metabolic rate, daily calorie expenditure, and other data to help you decide what's right for you. Regardless, you need to be 100 percent aware of all the foods you eat—the calories, the protein, the carbs, the fat. You need to maintain awareness of the calories burned from fasted cardio, Weight Chaining, and hyperactive ADL and IADL. From there, every decision needs to be contemplated using the cost-benefit analysis to help you make the heavy-handed beneficial choices in eating, exercise, and life.

CHAPTER 28
The Final Chapter: Not the End but the Beginning

Now you're ready to tear shit up! You're going to rock this motha-fucka like a Richter 9.0 earthquake!

You now have the tools, the knowledge, and the tricks of the trade professional bodybuilders use to achieve unreal fat-burning results. You are about to unleash hell on your body fat and incinerate it at a cataclysmic pace. Time to change your ways. Time to move. Time to fast. Time to mold your body composition into future you. Dreamed and imagined you. The you who conquers your future goals and ages successfully in place.

It is in our nature to do less to get more, which works against us when it comes to body composition. Or does it? Maybe getting lean and staying lean is possible with the same mindset or thoughts; just change the variables.

How? you say. Think about it. It's in our nature to do less to get more. So to be *less sedentary*, become *more* active. To eat *less*, metabolize *more* body fat! See? It is all a matter of perspective.

You have the power to do anything if your thoughts and actions support your dreams.

What you focus on comes true in the present and the future. Screw the past. Forget all the shit that has led you to this point, and focus on the now. Focus on how you want to look, feel, and live in the present. Never stop imagining your lean, light, and agile body. Believe in yourself, believe in the process, and take massive action. Believe that future you is inevitable and coming soon! Because it is.

Change the variables . . . change the results!

Change your beliefs.

Change your mindset.

Choose your thoughts.

Where you stare, energy penetrates, and outcomes reverberate.

Focus on the win.

Minimize regret.

Execute the plan.

Do not compromise.

And never stop . . . never.

At all costs, tune out the naysayers. Which there will be. Some kind of diabolical force shows its ugly head when people see you motivated and changing. They will become either inspired or jealous and subconsciously say, do, or try to derail you, sabotage your transformation, or put doubt in your thoughts. Sadly, the latter is what you will be dealing with, and it will include your closest loved ones, family, and friends. Don't be mad at them; it is human nature to be either inspired or jealous when witnessing physique changes. You control you. Nobody else can. You will need to stay firm in your resolve, focus on the prize, and stay true to the plan, all the while maintaining positive relationships with those you want in your life and avoiding the ones you don't.

This is your life we are talking about here, and life is short. This plan is meant to be implemented forever. No more yo-yo dieting and massive fluctuations in your body composition. This is the end of that absurdity.

Okay, time to stop talking about it.

It is time to do the work.

"Let's do this!"

Eat OBESE to be OBESE.
Eat LEAN to be LEAN.

It's not rocket science!

The End

BONUS
12 Dieting Facts

1. Fasting is healthy. Starving people are lean compared to people who overeat. Look at what happens to contestants on the TV show *Survivor*, or what people look like in countries short on food. Deprivation of calories and/or carbs and fat is the path to treat obesity.
2. Fat bodies will look smooth and plump until all the fat outside their lean bodies is burned off or metabolized.
3. If it wiggles, shakes, and jiggles, it's fat! Muscle and lean body tissue are solid and firm.
4. No amount of exercise will lead to a lean physique if the nutrition profile doesn't support fat burning. You must prepare your body for fat burning by *putting your body into a State of fat burning*.
5. If you consume more calories than your body metabolizes, the excess calories will be stored as body fat in most cases.
6. It is *not* easy to gain muscle.
7. It is *too* easy to gain body fat.
8. The more muscle you have, the higher your basal metabolic rate and therefore the easier to stay lean and burn body fat.
9. Gaining muscle or lean body mass should be every man's, woman's, and youth's goal in the quest for health and wellness. Lean muscle equals increased strength, increased metabolism, enhanced immunity, injury prevention, fall prevention, increased work output, and increased productivity.
10. Preventing body fat storage should be every man's, woman's, and youth's focus when consuming a meal. Focus should be on portion sizes, BV of protein, GI of carbs, and fat content.
11. Fasting is healthy and sometimes necessary, but it must be done in a safe and healthy way.
12. It is virtually impossible to metabolize body fat in a hyperglycemic state.

BONUS KISS Tips

1. Eat the same foods for your daily fasting and fat-burning regime.
2. Drink water to stay hydrated.
3. Coffee is king, but espresso is better. Due to the lack of a paper filter, espresso retains the natural healthy oils and minerals. Cold-press coffee is kinder to sensitive stomachs.
4. Stay busy! It keeps the mind occupied and thoughts focused.
5. Food prep is key to successful weight loss, health, and wellness.
6. Avoid eating out until your weight loss journey is complete and the maintenance phase ensues.
7. Avoid settings of temptation.
8. Do not deviate from your daily meal plan.
9. Stay motivated. Stay disciplined. Stay focused!
10. You must do the work to get paid or rewarded.
11. When in doubt, eat protein or fibrous vegetables.
12. When bored, move and don't stop until you've got something to do. The *EXER* in EXERLEAN equals *move*.
13. Listen to music during weightlifting. Watch the news, listen to an audiobook, or read a book during machine cardio.
14. Go to bed early to avoid late-evening snacking. Wake up early to have more time.
15. Know that your family, friends, and closest loved ones will likely not be your allies in your weight loss journey. Ignore them but love them anyway.
16. Aim to be around positive forces that bolster your ability to succeed and keep you motivated.
17. Keep a dumbbell set in your living room for a quick weight training session if needed. Ask your boss if a dumbbell set can be available for employee use during breaks.
18. Stretch in bed before going to sleep and when waking up.
19. Keep lean chicken, beef, turkey, or pork jerky on hand for meal emergencies.
20. Keep 40 grams of whey or soy isolate protein powder in a shaker on hand for meal emergencies.

Glossary

Chaining: EXERLEAN designer workout protocol, designed by John Blade. The *Weight Chaining* protocol works the body frontside to backside, or anterior chain to posterior chain. This format of weight training leaves the body in a heightened state of extension, leading to improved posture and overall functional stability.

EXERLEAN: "EXER" …for exercise or action; and "LEAN" …for everything lean: lean eating, lean foods, and having a lean body composition. The two together lead to maximal health, wellness, and build the foundation for aging and longevity. You cannot have one without the other and achieve ultimate awesomeness. EXER+LEAN=EXERLEAN: The Obesity Cure.

Healthstyle: The daily routine, schedule, agenda, habits, and behaviors that dictate your present and future status in maintaining a healthy body weight, body fat composition, physical activity and exercise level, work productivity, play, eating, and sleeping.

Sweet Blood: The state post carbohydrate consumption when the glucose in the blood is high, therefor most likely…sweet to the taste. It's a metaphor for hyperglycemia/high blood sugar and literally "sweet blood."

The State: The maximal setup of blood sugar levels, glycogen depletion, nitrogen retention, and protein loading, which creates the physiologic state of rapid maximal body fat thermogenesis…or FATBURNING!

Total Body Fat Incinerator: The TBFI…is a diet protocol designed by John Blade, the master of getting ripped to the gills. Total Body Fat Incinerator takes the power of The State and delivers it in a diet protocol for you to literally…incinerate your body fat. Ignite your internal Total Body Fat Incinerator and it will do just that…all you must do is turn it on by coding it to enter *The STATE*.

References

A "sleep 101" program for college students improves sleep hygiene knowledge and reduces maladaptive beliefs about sleep - pubmed. (2015). PubMed. https://pubmed.ncbi.nlm.nih.gov/25268924/

About – glycemic index. (2021). The University of Syndney: Glycemic Index Research and GI News. https://glycemicindex.com/about-gi/

Adinoff, B. (2004). Neurobiologic processes in drug reward and addiction. *Harvard Review of Psychiatry, 12*(6), 305–320. https://doi.org/10.1080/10673220490910844

Alan goldhamer, dc: Water fasting—the clinical effectiveness of rebooting your body. (2014). PubMed Central (PMC). https://www.ncbi.nlm.nih.gov/pmc/articles/PMC4684131/

Amino acids and immune function - pubmed. (2007). PubMed. https://pubmed.ncbi.nlm.nih.gov/17403271/

Amino acids and their significance for fat burning. (2021). http://www.aminoacid-studies.com. https://www.aminoacid-studies.com/areas-of-use/fat-burning.html

Amino acids: Effects, studies and tips. (2021). aminosaeuren.org. https://amino-acid.org/

Amino acids: Medlineplus medical encyclopedia. (2021). https://medlineplus.gov/ency/article/002222.htm

Baker, J. S., Davies, B., Cooper, S. M., Wong, D. P., Buchan, D. S., & Kilgore, L. (2013). Strength and body composition changes in recreationally strength-trained individuals: Comparison of one versus three sets resistance-training programmes. *BioMed Research International, 2013*, 1–6. https://doi.org/10.1155/2013/615901

Benefits of exercise. (2021). https://medlineplus.gov/benefitsofexercise.html

Benefits of glutamine: When to supplement. (2013, February 26). Bodybuilding.com. https://www.bodybuilding.com/content/all-about-glutamine-your-expert-guide.html

Benefits of physical activity. (2021, April 5). Centers for Disease Control and Prevention. https://www.cdc.gov/physicalactivity/basics/pa-health/index.htm

Biological value - wikipedia. (2021). https://en.wikipedia.org/wiki/Biological_value

Blade, J. (2001). *Fuel* [Essay]. John Blade.

Branched-chain amino acid supplementation promotes survival and supports cardiac and skeletal muscle mitochondrial biogenesis in middle-aged mice - pubmed. (2010). PubMed. https://pubmed.ncbi.nlm.nih.gov/20889128/

Carbohydrates, insulin overload, metabolic syndrome, and the glycemic index of food. (2011). The Longevity Institute. http://www.longevinst.org/nlt/GI.htm

CE International. (2018). *The diet revolution: neuroprotective & disease-modifying effects* [Continuing Education for Healthcare Professionals].

Centers for Disease Control and Prevention. (2020, November 17). *The health effects of overweight and obesity | healthy weight, nutrition, and physical activity | cdc.* CDC. https://www.cdc.gov/healthy-weight/effects/index.html

Chick, H., Boas-Fixsen, M., Hutchinson, J., & Jackson, H. (1935). The biological value of proteins. *Biochemical Journal, 29*(7), 1712–1719. https://doi.org/10.1042/bj0291712

Circuit training - wikipedia. (2021). https://en.wikipedia.org/wiki/Circuit_training

Classical conditioning - wikipedia. (2021). https://en.wikipedia.org/wiki/Classical_conditioning

Clinical guidelines on the identification, evaluation, and treatment of overweight and obesity in adults: the evidence report [PDF]. (1999). Obesity Education Initiative: National Institutes of Health. https://www.nhlbi.nih.gov/files/docs/guidelines/ob_gdlns.pdf

Cost–benefit analysis - wikipedia. (2021). https://en.wikipedia.org/wiki/Cost–benefit_analysis

Creating an active america together. (2020, September 17). Centers for Disease Control and Prevention. https://www.cdc.gov/physicalactivity/activepeoplehealthynation/about-active-people-healthy-nation.html

Current sports medicine reports. (2012). LWW. https://journals.lww.com/acsm-csmr/Fulltext/2012/07000/Resistance_Training_is_Medicine___Effects_of.13.aspx

Degrees of freedom (mechanics) - wikipedia. (2021). https://en.wikipedia.org/wiki/Degrees_of_freedom_(mechanics)

Dickerson, R. (2016). Nitrogen balance and protein requirements for critically ill older patients. *Nutrients, 8*(4), 226. https://doi.org/10.3390/nu8040226

Dietary fats explained: Medlineplus medical encyclopedia. (2021). https://medlineplus.gov/ency/patientinstructions/000104.htm

Do nitric oxide supplements work? an evidence-based review - legion athletics. (2015, April 26). Legion Athletics. https://legionathletics.com/nitric-oxide-supplements-science/

Drop in both insulin and leptin needed for fat burning to occur - diabetes. (2018). Diabetes. https://www.diabetes.co.uk/news/2018/jan/drop-in-both-insulin-and-leptin-needed-for-fat-burning-to-occur-90969878.html

Drop set - wikipedia. (2021). https://en.wikipedia.org/wiki/Drop_set

Eccentric training - wikipedia. (2021). https://en.wikipedia.org/wiki/Eccentric_training

Exercise: 7 benefits of regular physical activity. (2019). Mayo Clinic. https://www.mayoclinic.org/healthy-lifestyle/fitness/in-depth/exercise/art-20048389

Fasting: The history, pathophysiology and complications. (1982). PubMed Central (PMC). https://www.ncbi.nlm.nih.gov/pmc/articles/PMC1274154/

Fat: The facts. (n.d.). nhs.uk. https://www.nhs.uk/live-well/eat-well/different-fats-nutrition/

5 health benefits of nitric oxide supplements. (2018). Healthline. https://www.healthline.com/nutrition/nitric-oxide-supplements

Forbes, G. B., & Drenick, E. J. (1979). Loss of body nitrogen on fasting. *The American Journal of Clinical Nutrition, 32*(8), 1570–1574. https://doi.org/10.1093/ajcn/32.8.1570

Formation of amino acids from nh3 /no2, co2 and h2o: Implications for the prebiotic origin of biomolecules - pubmed. (2015). PubMed. https://pubmed.ncbi.nlm.nih.gov/26443411/

Free will - wikipedia. (2021). https://en.wikipedia.org/wiki/Free_will

Ghrelin - wikipedia. (2021). https://en.wikipedia.org/wiki/Ghrelin

Glycemic index - wikipedia. (2021). https://en.wikipedia.org/wiki/Glycemic_index

Glycemic index for 60+ foods. (2020). Harvard Health Publishing: Harvard Medical School. https://www.health.harvard.edu/diseases-and-conditions/glycemic-index-and-glycemic-load-for-100-foods

Glycogen - wikipedia. (2021). https://en.wikipedia.org/wiki/Glycogen

Goal setting theory of motivation. (2021). https://www.managementstudyguide.com/goal-setting-theory-motivation.htm

Gravity hurts (so good) | science mission directorate. (2001). NASA SCIENCE: SHARE THE SCIENCE. https://science.nasa.gov/science-news/science-at-nasa/2001/ast02aug_1

Harris, J., Engberg, J., & Castle, N. (2018). Obesity and intensive staffing needs of nursing home residents. *Geriatric Nursing, 39*(6), 696–701. https://doi.org/10.1016/j.gerinurse.2018.05.006

Hatfield, F. C., PhD. (2016). *Fitness: The Complete Guide* (9th ed.). International Sports Sciences Association. https://doi.org/https://books.issaonline.com/product/cft

Health effects of a diet that mimics fasting. (2015, August 19). National Institutes of Health (NIH). https://www.nih.gov/news-events/nih-research-matters/health-effects-diet-mimics-fasting

Health risks of an inactive lifestyle. (2017). https://medlineplus.gov/healthrisksofaninactivelifestyle.html

Healthy people - healthy people 2020. (2020, December 14). Centers for Disease Control and Prevention. https://www.cdc.gov/nchs/healthy_people/hp2020.htm

High and low biological value protein foods. (2008). eufic: food facts for health choices. https://www.eufic.org/en/whats-in-food/article/the-basics-proteins

High-protein diet - wikipedia. (2021). https://en.wikipedia.org/wiki/High-protein_diet

Hindawi. (2012). *Sedentary behaviors, weight, and health and disease risks.* https://www.hindawi.com/journals/jobe/2012/852743/

Hindle, K., Whitcomb, T., Briggs, W., & Hong, J. (2012). Proprioceptive neuromuscular facilitation (pnf): Its mechanisms and effects on range of motion and muscular function. *Journal of Human Kinetics, 31*(2012), 105–113. https://doi.org/10.2478/v10078-012-0011-y

Hoffman, J., & Falvo, M. (2004). Protein - Which is Best?. *Journal of sports science & medicine*, (3), 118–130.

How can bcaas boost muscle building? (2014). Shape. https://www.shape.com/healthy-eating/diet-tips/ask-diet-doctor-essential-amino-acids

How to load up on protein to lose weight. (2014, November 12). Women's Health. https://www.womenshealthmag.com/weight-loss/a19982570/how-to-eat-more-protein/

How to use the glycemic index. (2021). WebMD. https://www.webmd.com/diabetes/guide/glycemic-index-good-versus-bad-carbs

Hunger - wikipedia. (2021). https://en.wikipedia.org/wiki/Hunger

Hunger (physiology) - wikipedia. (2021). https://en.wikipedia.org/wiki/Hunger_(physiology)

Increasing lean mass and strength: A comparison of high frequency strength training to lower frequency strength training - pubmed. (2016). PubMed. https://pubmed.ncbi.nlm.nih.gov/27182422/

INR (Institute for Natural Resources. (2020). *The Science of Fat & Sugar* (8th ed.). INR (Institute for Natural Resources).

Institute for Natural Resources (INR). (2018). *Obesity, Diet, & Behavior* (4th ed.) [Continuing Education Booklet for healthcare professionals]. INR (Institute for Natural Resources.

Intermittent fasting - wikipedia. (2021). https://en.wikipedia.org/wiki/Intermittent_fasting

Intermittent fasting and human metabolic health. (2015). PubMed Central (PMC). https://www.ncbi.nlm.nih.gov/pmc/articles/PMC4516560/

Intermittent fasting: The science of going without | cmaj. (2013). https://www.cmaj.ca/content/185/9/E363

Intermittent fasting: The science of going without. (2013). PubMed Central (PMC). https://www.ncbi.nlm.nih.gov/pmc/articles/PMC3680567/

International tables of glycemic index and glycemic load values: 2008 | diabetes care. (2008). https://care.diabetesjournals.org/content/31/12/2281

ISSA. (2021). *Understanding and using the overload principle | issa*. https://www.issaonline.com/blog/index.cfm/2019/understanding-and-using-the-overload-principle

Kava, R. (2016). *Obesity: what's metabolic rate got to do with it?* American Council on Science and Health. https://www.acsh.org/news/2016/10/15/obesity-whats-metabolic-rate-got-do-it-10306

L-carnitine - a review of benefits, side effects and dosage. (2021). Healthline. https://www.healthline.com/nutrition/l-carnitine

Lee, W. H., R.Ph, Ph.D. (1989). *Concentrated Fat Burners* [Booklet]. Dr. William H. Lee.

Leptin - wikipedia. (2021). https://en.wikipedia.org/wiki/Leptin

Li, Z., Liu, H., Yin, Z., & Chen, K. (2019). Muscle synergy alteration of human during walking with lower limb exoskeleton. *Frontiers in Neuroscience, 12.* https://doi.org/10.3389/fnins.2018.01050

Long-term services and supports - aarp fact sheet [PDF]. (2019). AARP. https://www.aarp.org/content/dam/aarp/ppi/2019/08/long-term-services-and-supports.doi.10.26419-2Fppi.00079.001.pdf

Maslows hierarchy of needs theory. (2021). https://www.management-studyguide.com/maslows-hierarchy-needs-theory.htm

Moore, D. R., & Soeters, P. B. (2020). The biological value of protein. In *The importance of nutrition as an integral part of disease management* (pp. 39–51). S. Karger AG. https://doi.org/10.1159/000382000

Motor coordination - wikipedia. (2021). https://en.wikipedia.org/wiki/Motor_coordination

Muscle growth. (2012). amino acid studies. https://aminoacidstudies.org/muscle-growth/

N. Gearhardt, A., Davis, C., Kuschner, R., & D. Brownell, K. (2011). The addiction potential of hyperpalatable foods. *Current Drug Abuse Reviewse, 4*(3), 140–145. https://doi.org/10.2174/1874473711104030140

Nad+ biosynthesis, aging, and disease. (2018). PubMed Central (PMC). https://www.ncbi.nlm.nih.gov/pmc/articles/PMC5795269/

Nchs pressroom - 2000 fact sheet - u.s. nursing homes profiled in a new report. (2006). CDC. https://www.cdc.gov/nchs/pressroom/00facts/nurshome.htm

Nitrogen balance - wikipedia. (2021). https://en.wikipedia.org/wiki/Nitrogen_balance

Nitrogen balance. (1947). *Journal of the American Medical Association, 133*(4), 247. https://doi.org/10.1001/jama.1947.02880040033010

Nitrogen balance: The key to muscle growth. (2005, May 17). Bodybuilding.com. https://www.bodybuilding.com/fun/drobson75.htm

Nursing home data compendium 2015 [PDF]. (2016). Department of Health & Human Services CMS. https://www.cms.gov/Medicare/Provider-Enrollment-and-Certification/CertificationandComplianc/Downloads/nursinghomedatacompendium_508-2015.pdf

Peptide yy - wikipedia. (2021). https://en.wikipedia.org/wiki/Peptide_YY

Pesta, D. H., & Samuel, V. T. (2014). A high-protein diet for reducing body fat: Mechanisms and possible caveats. *Nutrition & Metabolism, 11*(1), 53. https://doi.org/10.1186/1743-7075-11-53

Protein digestibility corrected amino acid score - wikipedia. (2021). https://en.wikipedia.org/wiki/Protein_Digestibility_Corrected_Amino_Acid_Score

Protein in diet: Medlineplus medical encyclopedia. (2021). https://medlineplus.gov/ency/article/002467.htm

Quinn, E. (2019). *Get pumped with supersets in weight training*. Verywell Fit. https://www.verywellfit.com/what-is-a-superset-3120397

Rational choice theory - wikipedia. (2021). https://en.wikipedia.org/wiki/Rational_choice_theory

Regret (decision theory) - wikipedia. (2021). https://en.wikipedia.org/wiki/Regret_(decision_theory)

Sarcopenia and frailty in elderly trauma patients. (2015). PubMed Central (PMC). https://www.ncbi.nlm.nih.gov/pmc/articles/PMC5215219/

Sarcopenia, sarcopenic obesity, and functional impairments in older adults: National health and nutrition examination surveys 1999-2004 - pubmed. (2015). PubMed. https://pubmed.ncbi.nlm.nih.gov/26472145/

Sarcopenia, sarcopenic obesity and inflammation: Results from the 1999-2004 national health and nutrition examination survey - pubmed. (2016). PubMed. https://pubmed.ncbi.nlm.nih.gov/27091774/

Sedentary behavior and health outcomes: An overview of systematic reviews - pubmed. (2014). PubMed. https://pubmed.ncbi.nlm.nih.gov/25144686/

Sedentary behavior: Emerging evidence for a new health risk. (2010). PubMed Central (PMC). https://www.ncbi.nlm.nih.gov/pmc/articles/PMC2996155/

Sedentary behavior: emerging evidence for a new health risk [Volume 85, issue 12, P1138-1141]. (2010, December 1). Mayo Clinic Proceedings. https://www.mayoclinicproceedings.org/article/S0025-6196(11)60368-6/fulltext

Sedentary behavior, physical activity and cardiorespiratory fitness on leukocyte telomere length. (2016). PubMed Central (PMC). https://www.ncbi.nlm.nih.gov/pmc/articles/PMC5209646/

Sedentary behavior: Target for change, challenge to assess - pubmed. (2012). PubMed. https://pubmed.ncbi.nlm.nih.gov/25089191/

Sedentary behaviour and risk of all-cause, cardiovascular and cancer mortality, and incident type 2 diabetes: A systematic review and dose response meta-analysis - pubmed. (2017). PubMed. https://pubmed.ncbi.nlm.nih.gov/29589226/

Selected long-term care statistics - family caregiver alliance. (2021). https://www.caregiver.org/resource/selected-long-term-care-statistics/

Self-actualization - wikipedia. (2021). https://en.wikipedia.org/wiki/Self-actualization

Six degrees of freedom - wikipedia. (2021). https://en.wikipedia.org/wiki/Six_degrees_of_freedom

6 vein-popping reasons to use nitric oxide supplements! (2010, May 23). Bodybuilding.com. https://www.bodybuilding.com/content/6-vein-popping-reasons-to-use-nitric-oxide-supplements.html

Sports periodization - wikipedia. (2021). https://en.wikipedia.org/wiki/Sports_periodization

Strength training improves body image and physical activity behaviors among midlife and older rural women. (2013). PubMed Central (PMC). https://www.ncbi.nlm.nih.gov/pmc/articles/PMC4354895/

Strength training in children and adolescents: Raising the bar for young athletes? - pubmed. (2009). PubMed. https://pubmed.ncbi.nlm.nih.gov/23015875/

Strengthening the immune system. (2021). amino-acid.org. https://amino-acid.org/strengthening-the-immune-system/

Support. (2013). *Glycemicindex* [PDF]. https://extension.oregonstate.edu/sites/default/files/documents/1/glycemicindex.pdf

The benefits of amino acids: Why we take bcaas. (2014, September 10). Bodybuilding.com. https://www.bodybuilding.com/content/bcaas-the-many-benefits-of-amino-acids.html

The effects of protein and amino acid supplementation on performance and training adaptations during ten weeks of resistance training - pubmed. (2006). PubMed. https://pubmed.ncbi.nlm.nih.gov/16937979/

The intensity and effects of strength training in the elderly. (2011). PubMed Central (PMC). https://www.ncbi.nlm.nih.gov/pmc/articles/PMC3117172/

The most important amino acid for athletes? (2019). Dr. Axe. https://draxe.com/nutrition/l-carnitine/

The role of leptin and ghrelin in the regulation of food intake and body weight in humans: A review - pubmed. (2007). PubMed. https://pubmed.ncbi.nlm.nih.gov/17212793/

The role of peptide yy in appetite regulation and obesity - pubmed. (2009). PubMed. https://pubmed.ncbi.nlm.nih.gov/19064614/

The therapeutic benefits of gravity in space and on earth. (2008). PubMed Central (PMC). https://www.ncbi.nlm.nih.gov/pmc/articles/PMC2577396/

To fast or not to fast. (2019, November 22). NIH News in Health. https://newsinhealth.nih.gov/2019/12/fast-or-not-fast

Tocino-Smith, J., Msc. (2019, April 19). *What is locke's goal setting theory of motivation*. PositivePsychology.com. https://positivepsychology.com/goal-setting-theory/

Too much sitting: The population-health science of sedentary behavior. (2010). PubMed Central (PMC). https://www.ncbi.nlm.nih.gov/pmc/articles/PMC3404815/

top 10 benefits of amino acid supplements - june 2021. (2017). https://thefeed.com/blogs/news/10-benefits-of-amino-acid-supplements

U.S. Department of Health and Human Services. (2021). *Overweight and obesity*. Healthy People 2030. https://health.gov/healthypeople/objectives-and-data/browse-objectives/overweight-and-obesity

U.S. Department of Veterans Affairs. (2021). *Va.gov | veterans affairs*. https://www.va.gov/WHOLEHEALTHLIBRARY/tools/glycemic-index.asp

Varney, S. (2021). *Rising obesity puts strain on nursing homes*. Kaiser Family Foundation. https://khn.org/news/rising-obesity-puts-strain-on-nursing-homes-2/

Vitamins and minerals - helpguide.org [A Harvard Health Article]. (2021). HelpGuide.org. https://www.helpguide.org/harvard/vitamins-and-minerals.htm

Warburton, D. E. (2006). Health benefits of physical activity: The evidence. *Canadian Medical Association Journal, 174*(6), 801–809. https://doi.org/10.1503/cmaj.051351

Water fasting: Benefits, weight loss, and how to do it [Newsletter]. (2018). Medical News Today. https://www.medicalnewstoday.com/articles/319835

Wechsler, J., Wenzel, H., Swobodnik, W., Ditschuneit, H., & Ditschuneit, H. (1984). *Nitrogen balance studies during modified fasting - pubmed*. PubMed. https://pubmed.ncbi.nlm.nih.gov/6514657/

What are amino acid supplements | women's health. (2017, November 9). Women's Health. https://www.womenshealthmag.com/fitness/a19962078/amino-acid-workout-boost/

Whey protein, amino acids may boost fat loss. (2012, December 12). WebMD. https://www.webmd.com/diet/news/20121212/whey-amino-acids-fat-loss

Other Resources

1. https://www.ncbi.nlm.nih.gov/pmc/articles/PMC3905294/
2. Per https://www.big5sportinggoods.com/store/
3. *NIH News in Health* post "Counting Carbs?: Understanding Glycemic Index and Glycemic Load" from December 2012, which you can find online. A great free resource for the glycemic index can be found in the American Diabetes Association (ADA) *Diabetes Care* article "International Tables of Glycemic Index and Glycemic load Values: 2008"; see the first supplemental table. If this list is too huge, then under the Figures & Tables tab is a condensed glycemic index table and link to a PDF to download. Also see the tabs Article, Supplemental Material, and Info & Metrics.

Referrals

Book Editor : Christina Roth Editorial

Cover Design: George Stevens G-Sharp Design LLC

EXERLEAN artwork,

99designs artist : "ardifa"

99designs artist : "faceless"

99designs artist : "NocrapDesigns"

99designs artist : "TONG"

Total Body Fat Incinerator artwork,

99designs artist : "Andre Filipe Kautzmann, AKA Mr. Kautzmann"

99designs artist : "Romulo Sudario Jr. AKA Bodski Meg"

Weight Chaining artwork,

99designs artist : "Dee Junt"

99designs artist : "LuckyOne"

99designs artist : "SEMOX"

99designs artist : "huma_maira"

99designs artist : "brainfox"

About the Author

Credentials

John Blade is a well credentialed professional, including being a national registered, board certified, and state licensed Occupational Therapist (OTRL). He holds certifications in Aging in Place (CAPS) through the National Association of Home Builders (NAHB), is a certified personal trainer (CPT) through the International Sport Strength Association (ISSA), holds certificates for both Advance Cardiac Life Support & Basic Life Support (ACLS & BLS)

History

John has been competing in the sport of bodybuilding since 1997 when he completed his first competition, The National Physique Committee (NPC) IRONMAN Naturally. He has since competed in many more shows over the years. Prior to finishing OT school, he was a Gold's Gym personal trainer, and helped many clients achieve amazing transformations.

John not only competed in bodybuilding shows, but also power lifting competitions. All the while competing in bodybuilding and powerlifting competitions, John spent many years training martial arts in depth with Sifu Joseph Simonet and Addy Hernandez of Ki Fighting Concepts.

Other Interests

John has been a Bitcoin miner since its release in 2009. Due to an overwhelming amount of people wanting information on Bitcoin mining and Bitcoin in general; he wrote a book on the subjects to help people become Bitcoin miners themselves, or invest in other Bitcoin and cryptocurrency investments if they so choose. The book is titled, "The Bitcoin

Capital of the World," He enjoys computer technology, builds his own gaming/video editing powerhouse computers, and when able enjoys PC gaming, video creation and editing, and digital music composition.

My Mission

I...John Blade, like many others on this earth know many things, and some with absolute precision expertise, or enlightenment. If there is one thing John Blade has the expertise, wherewithal, and knowledge on is to get fricken ripped...ripped to the gills. Total Body Fat Incineration is easy if you have the fortitude and discipline to follow the EXERLEAN program. As an OT in the hospital, I help people get better, to move better, to feel better, and ultimately to GET OUT of the hospital. Over the years, my observation of the patient population (people that need to be hospitalized) hold one dominating trait above all others...OBESITY. My Mission...the end the obesity epidemic by giving people the necessary knowledge and tools to make their own transformation possible.

www.ingramcontent.com/pod-product-compliance
Lightning Source LLC
Chambersburg PA
CBHW051616010526
44107CB00042B/1493/J